PHARMACY RESEARCH

A How-To Guide for Students, Residents, and New Practitioners

American Pharmacists Association
Books and Electronic Products
Mission Statement

Our mission is to provide engaging resources for the profession to advance patient care and improve medication use.

We will achieve this by

- Providing the profession with authoritative content
- Offering products that enhance patient care, practice management, and leadership in the profession
- Delivering innovative solutions for the market
- Serving our members with the tools needed for continuing professional development

Notice

PHARMACY RESEARCH

A How-To Guide for Students, Residents, and New Practitioners

Rosalyn Padiyara Vellurattil, PharmD, CDE
Assistant Dean of Academic Affairs
Clinical Associate Professor
Department of Pharmacy Systems, Outcomes, and Policy
University of Illinois at Chicago College of Pharmacy
Chicago, Illinois

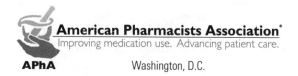

American Pharmacists Association®
Improving medication use. Advancing patient care.
APhA
Washington, D.C.

Acquiring Editor: Julian Graubart
Editor: Nancy Tarleton Landis
Managing Editor: Janan Sarwar
Proofreaders: Publications Professionals LLC
Indexing: Suzanne Peake
Cover Design: Mariam Bederu, APhA Integrated Design and Production Center
Composition: Circle Graphics

Published by the American Pharmacists Association, 2215 Constitution Avenue, NW,
Washington, DC 20037-2985

www.pharmacist.com www.pharmacylibrary.com

To comment on this book via e-mail, send your message to the publisher at aphabooks@
aphanet.org.

Library of Congress Cataloging-in-Publication-Data
Vellurattil, Rosalyn Padiyara, author.
 Pharmacy research : a how-to guide for students, residents, and new practitioners / Rosalyn
Padiyara Vellurattil.
    p. ; cm.
Includes bibliographical references.
ISBN 978-1-58212-241-0
I. American Pharmacists Association, issuing body. II. Title.
[DNLM: 1. Biomedical Research—methods. 2. Pharmacy. 3. Mentors. 4. Research Design.
QV 20.5]
RM301.27
615.1072'4—dc23

2015024910

How to Order This book
Online: www.pharmacist.com/shop
By phone: 800-878-0729 (770-280-0085 from outside the United States)
VISA®, MasterCard®, and American Express® cards accepted

For my mother

Contents

Preface

Performing research in pharmacy is a necessary and essential component of the profession. In fact, research is a necessary and essential component of all health care professions. No discipline can thrive without creating new knowledge to meet existing or emerging challenges. The research that is performed is not only of importance to the researchers conducting it but of great value to patients, practice, education, the medical community, and society at large. The use of systematic research processes enables us to investigate and test methods that can improve quality and best practices in health care.

In fact, if you think about it, research is quite a noble and selfless way of giving back to your profession. Does that mean you have to be the most seasoned expert in order to make a contribution? No, not by any means! However, like any inexperienced person entering a new field, all novice researchers must undergo proper training and education. In the world of pharmacy today, where opportunities for employment and residency are extremely competitive, research experience sets you apart from other new graduates and provides you with an additional skill set that increases your marketability. Think about that for a second. You are gaining experience and skills that not all of your peers possess, that can help you attain career opportunities and satisfaction and allow you to make a meaningful difference in the world. How is that not a win–win situation?

Having performed research for a number of years, and having worked with both pharmacy students and residents on various research projects, I became convinced that a resource geared toward learning the basics of research would be extremely useful to budding researchers. The goal of this book is to provide pharmacy students, residents, and new practitioners with an introduction to research methods and a foundation on which individual research practices can be built. The book offers a simple, step-by-step guide with practical tips and advice on the phases of completing a pharmacy-based research project. Each chapter details a phase in the research process and discusses the steps for moving to the next level. Included, too, are personal reflections that provide insight into the nature of mentor–mentee relationships. Students, new graduates, residents, and any practitioners needing basic training in research fundamentals will find this a valuable resource.

About the Author

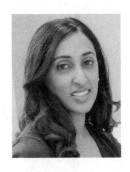

Rosalyn Padiyara Vellurattil, PharmD, CDE, is Assistant Dean of Academic Affairs, University of Illinois at Chicago College of Pharmacy, and a Clinical Associate Professor in the Department of Pharmacy Systems, Outcomes, and Policy. Previously, she was Director of Capstone and Milemarker Experiences at Chicago State University College of Pharmacy. She received her Doctor of Pharmacy degree from the University of Illinois at Chicago and completed a specialty residency in primary care with a focus on education from Midwestern University Chicago College of Pharmacy.

Dr. Vellurattil has served as an educator, researcher, and mentor to pharmacy students and residents in the academic setting since 2004. Her research interests have included pharmacist-managed ambulatory care services and outcomes, postgraduate training, and pharmacy education. She has presented her work at several national professional society meetings and published in a variety of peer-reviewed journals.

CHAPTER 1

Where Do I Begin?

Learning Objectives

1. Identify the initial steps in beginning a research project.
2. Develop a research question.
3. Define the roles of the study investigators.
4. Evaluate available funding opportunities.

Key Terms

- Research
- Research question/hypothesis
- Study investigators
- Mentor–mentee relationship
- Funding

Research is formalized curiosity.
It is poking and prying with a purpose.
—Zora Neale Hurston

As a student, resident, or new practitioner with little exposure to research, you may be wondering where to start. The research process has many steps, but the first thing you should ask yourself is, What am I interested in researching? All research projects begin with a question (or hypothesis). Developing a research question is not always an easy task, but it begins with selecting a topic that interests you. What is your passion? Medication safety? Disease management? Pharmacy education? Are you most interested in laboratory or bench work? Clinical work? Social or behavioral work? What are you curious about? What do you hope to accomplish? Take a moment for self-reflection, and explore your personal research interests (Appendix A).

Types of Research in Pharmacy

Pharmacy research areas range from laboratory research to clinical research to survey and educational research. Laboratory research studies are conducted in the controlled environment of a research facility and may involve disciplines such as pharmacology/toxicology, pharmaceutics, drug discovery/medicinal chemistry, and immunology/biomedical sciences. Clinical research and survey research are population-based studies in human subjects. This type of research may involve areas such as global health, public policy, outcomes, protocol development, education, patient safety, and quality improvement/assurance. Educational research involves evaluation of teaching methods or student learning in a didactic or experiential setting, assessment of program outcomes, classroom dynamics, or faculty development.

Developing a Research Question

In developing your research question, you need to first select an area within the type of research that interests you. Take clinical research, for example. What is it about clinical research that interests you? Perhaps as a student you realized that you love the area of diabetes, or perhaps you work in a diabetes clinic and you wonder whether your patients who use Lantus (insulin glargine; sanofi-aventis) once daily fare just as well those who use it twice daily. Simply thinking about this question has given you an idea for your research. A list of potential research topic areas and questions (Appendix B) will help you get started brainstorming.

Study Investigators and Collaboration

Once you've decided what area of research interests you most and what your research question is going to be, one of your next tasks is to seek out an experienced mentor in that area who can help guide you in your research.

This can be fairly easy if you are a student, since you may know professors who work in your area of interest or perform research in that area. If you are a resident, you may consider working with the preceptor of one of your rotations. If you are a new practitioner, you may think of a professor or mentor with whom you interacted in the past or now work with as a collaborator. You may also want to work on your project with peers or colleagues who have similar interests. Consider enlisting the help of a statistician for data analysis. Your mentor, residency director, research program coordinator, or employer can provide guidance in this area and may be able to suggest someone. Involving the statistician early in the development of your project is beneficial so that statistical tests can be discussed from the very beginning. In these initial stages of developing a research project, you will be seeking and forming relationships with potential co-investigators.

Although research can be performed alone, it is most often performed by a team. Team members help share the workload, provide motivation, and share accountability in completing tasks. All teams have a lead investigator (also known as the principal investigator) and co-investigators. Every member of the team contributes a level of expertise, and all perspectives should be considered in the design and development of a project.

The Mentor–Mentee Relationship

Establishing a mentor–mentee relationship can be a rewarding experience, both professionally and personally, for all involved. Mentees can bring refreshing new perspective and motivation to a research project, while mentors provide the guidance, support, and inspiration that are essential. The relationship is built on mutual trust and respect for one another. It is a mentor's job to coach, challenge, and empower, and this in turn fosters trust, communication, and accountability on the mentee's part. Appendix C outlines the responsibilities of mentors and mentees in developing successful research relationships.

Obtaining Funding Resources

Funding is another factor to consider in developing a research project. Does your research require special equipment, tests, or preparatory tools? Do you plan to mail surveys to every household in your state? Do you want to be able to provide incentives or goodie bags to help recruit participants in your study? Will you be hiring any consultants or statisticians for the project? If you answer yes to any of these questions, then you should consider obtaining funding.

Funding can be sought internally or externally. For a first-time researcher, obtaining internal funding provides practical experience for obtaining larger external grants in the future. Does your university or institution provide grants that can be applied for to support research efforts? Does your mentor work with a professional organization that provides funding? Discuss with the mentor whether it is necessary or reasonable to obtain funding for your research. Pursuing funding opportunities is a great experience, regardless of whether the project ultimately is funded. The application process helps enhance your writing skills and provides you with useful feedback for pursuing funding in the future.

Completing a Research Project

It is often easy for students to join a mentor, preceptor, or faculty member's existing research project. This is a great way to volunteer and gain some research experience. The same opportunity exists for residents. Research projects require time, commitment, and perseverance. These demands will be problematic if you choose a project that does not interest you. A project of true interest to the researcher not only potentiates curiosity but also stimulates innovation. When you set out to seek answers to an existing problem or discover an existing gap, you have essentially developed a research question.

Additional Resources

1. Blessing JD, Forister JG, eds. *Introduction to Research and Medical Literature for Health Professionals.* 3rd ed. Burlington, MA: Jones and Bartlett Learning, LLC; 2013.
2. Jacobsen KH. *Introduction to Health Research Methods: A Practical Guide.* Sudbury, MA: Jones and Bartlett Learning, LLC; 2012.

Where to Begin Checklist

☐ Choose a research topic area

☐ Develop a research question

☐ Seek out a research mentor

☐ Choose your co-investigators and collaborators

☐ Consider working with a statistician

☐ Develop a plan for funding as necessary

CHAPTER 2

What Do I Need to Do to Get Started?

Learning Objectives

1. Perform a literature search.
2. Refine your research question.
3. Develop a research proposal and timeline.
4. Define your study design.
5. Differentiate between referencing formats.

Key Terms

- Literature search
- Research proposal
- Study design
- Timeline
- Referencing

> *Research is creating new knowledge.*
> *—Neil Armstrong*

Now that you have thought about a potential research question, it's time to refine that idea into something more concrete. Let's revisit the diabetes example. You are interested in determining whether your patients using

Lantus once daily fared just as well those using it twice daily. What do you do next?

You must conduct a literature search to determine what has been published on the topic. Your initial search may reveal that your research question has already been answered. Alternatively, you may find that the question has been answered but that more questions have arisen from that research, or that the question has not been answered at all.

Refining Your Research Question

It is important to critically evaluate the literature on your topic to refine your research idea into a question that is more specific and focused. Perhaps in your literature review you find that your topic has been looked at in the pediatric population but not in the obese adult population that you are interested in. You have now just refined your question to the following: Do obese adult patients with diabetes using Lantus once daily fare just as well using Lantus twice daily? How could you make this question more detailed? How could "fare just as well" be interpreted? Are there particular outcomes related to diabetes that you can include to make the question more specific? The question for you to answer as a researcher now has been refined and focused, as follows: Do obese adults patients with diabetes using Lantus once daily differ in fasting blood glucose outcomes from those using Lantus twice daily? Your literature search has helped refine the question; a gap exists in the currently available literature and your research will provide information for closing that gap.

As you perform your research, you may find that more questions arise that could be further researched. No need to worry—that is part of the research cycle. Research questions beget more research questions and provide further opportunities for you or others to investigate.

Research Proposals and Timelines

Your research plan should include developing a research proposal. This proposal becomes the framework when you are ready to begin developing your research manuscript. What is involved in developing a research proposal? You've already begun by developing a research question and performing an initial literature search. These steps are the basis for further developing background information on your topic and imparting to others the rationale for performing this research. Keep in mind that simply performing your research does not make it significant. It is your job to persuade anyone who comes across your topic to want to learn more about it, to be curious enough to continue reading. You must be convincing when writing both your proposal and your eventual manuscript. Make your audience understand the topic's importance and what its place in the literature will be.

A research proposal not only includes the background and significance of your topic; it also defines the purpose and objectives of your study, describes the methods by which you will conduct your study, and explains how you will collect results and what statistical methods you will use to analyze them (Appendix D). Also incorporated in the research proposal is a budget showing how you intend to use any funding you may have obtained.

A timeline is included to indicate when you anticipate completing the various steps of your research. Keep in mind that performing research is a lengthy process; things that may be beyond your control can occur and cause unintended delays. To help prevent this, begin by submitting an application for your proposed project to the appropriate institutional review board (IRB) early in the process, as you cannot begin your project until it is approved. As a resident, you have a yearlong time frame to conduct your project; make your submission to the IRB by the end of August or early September. For students, research time frames may vary from less than a year to more than a year. Early on, be sure to obtain guidance from your mentor as to what the expectations will be, and create a timeline accordingly. Appendix E provides an example of a research proposal.

Study Design

There are various types of study approaches that you may consider as you plan your research, from reviews or meta-analyses to correlational studies, case series, cross-sectional studies, cohort studies, experimental studies, and qualitative studies.[1,2] The intent of this chapter is not to review what these types of studies entail but rather to guide you in determining how to select your study design. If you need a refresher, the texts listed in the reference section of this chapter are great for beginners. You can also review statistics and drug literature evaluation references you may have used (or are currently using) while in pharmacy school.

Determining the study approach is the second step in the research process (Appendix F). In selecting an appropriate study design, you need to first ask yourself, Which study design is most appropriate for what I intend to study? Base your answer on the type of information you want to explore, and choose the study design according to the information you want to collect. Let's discuss this further by going back to the original diabetes example. You've determined that the objective you want to investigate is whether obese adult patients with diabetes using Lantus once daily differ in fasting blood glucose outcomes from those using Lantus twice daily. This information can be collected retrospectively, prospectively, or via survey. It can involve a single center or multiple centers. Since you are currently working in a diabetes clinic, you and your mentor decide the information can be best collected through retrospective chart review at your clinic as a pilot study. Since you've seen multiple patients using twice-daily dosing, you also have the ability to review their charts for outcomes over a defined period of time.

What protocol or procedures will you have your sample population follow? In designing the study, you will begin to develop a protocol on what the sample populations you are targeting will look like and what procedure they need to follow to minimize biases and confounding variables. In the example, you decide Sample A will be obese adult patients with diabetes using Lantus once daily, and Sample B will be obese adult patients with diabetes using Lantus twice daily. The outcome measures will be fasting blood glucose, 2-hour postprandial blood glucose, and A1c. You decide that both populations must check their blood glucose levels at least twice a day and must not be renally impaired. These specifications now become your inclusion and exclusion criteria for patients who would qualify for review.

Referencing Formats

As you begin writing your research proposal, format your references from the very beginning. If you plan to publish a research manuscript in the future, note that most journals use the American Medical Association (AMA) format. Journals may also follow the Uniform Requirements for Manuscripts Submitted to Biomedical Journals. You can learn more about the AMA style manual at http://www.amamanualofstyle.com/.

Your residency director (for residents) or research program coordinator/ director (for students) may have a preferred reference style for you to use, so check with that person at the outset. As time goes on and your manuscript continues to develop, you can change the formatting of your references according to the specific journal in which you want to publish. Visit the journal's website and search for the manuscript submission guidelines for authors. Details on the referencing format that the journal prefers will be provided there. Formatting your references early on will save you time later when you are ready to submit for publication.

Referencing Software

Depending on the topic you have chosen to research, you may find that there is an enormous amount of literature available or, in the opposite case, not enough. You may want to consider using referencing software for projects with a large number of references (e.g., 25 or more). There are various reference managers available. EndNote (http://endnote.com) and RefWorks (https://www.refworks.com) in particular are quite popular, but they are not free. You may want to first check with your mentor, preceptor, director, or institution to see if there is an institutional license you can use. For research with a large number of sources of information, reference managers are beneficial; the software will automatically reorganize and renumber the reference list as well as citations within the text when you make adjustments in your writing. There are a few free demonstration versions available online that you may want to try as well, such as Mendeley (www.mendeley.com), Qiqqa (www.qiqqa.com), and Zotero (www.zotero. org), but you may be limited to a certain number of references or storage on these versions.

Using referencing software is not mandatory. Since this may be the first time you are conducting and documenting research, do what you feel most comfortable with, whether that be manually adjusting references or using software. If the latter, be sure to give yourself enough time to become familiar with the product and test it. In considering a product to use, ask yourself, Is it compatible with my operating system? Are there screen shots or video tours available to view on the website? Reading reviews on Google or reviewing how-to videos on YouTube can help you decide to use or not use software.

References

1. Blessing JD, Forister JG, eds. *Introduction to Research and Medical Literature for Health Professionals.* 3rd ed. Burlington, MA: Jones and Bartlett Learning, LLC; 2013.
2. Jacobsen KH. *Introduction to Health Research Methods: A Practical Guide.* Sudbury, MA: Jones and Bartlett Learning, LLC; 2012.

Getting Started Checklist

☐ Perform a literature search

☐ Critically evaluate the literature search results to refine your research question

☐ Develop a research proposal (introduction, objectives, methods, references) and timeline to follow for the specified length of your project

☐ Implement your research timeline

☐ Determine your study design and include specifics on protocol/procedures within the research proposal

☐ Develop a plan for referencing

☐ Develop a plan using referencing software as necessary

CHAPTER 3

What Approvals Are Necessary?

Learning Objectives

1. Demonstrate knowledge of institutional review boards.
2. Determine which types of training your institution or employer requires you to undergo.
3. Develop an application according to the research you are conducting, applying your training and research principles to the application.
4. Create a curriculum vitae and continually refine it.

Key Terms

- Institutional review board
- Human subjects, informed consent, ethics training
- Curriculum vitae

Facts, and facts alone, are the foundation of science. . . . When one devotes oneself to experimental research it is in order to augment the sum of known facts, or to discover their mutual relations.
—*François Magendie*

Institutional review boards (IRBs) review and approve human subjects research, ensure that informed consent is documented, discuss whether ethical requirements have been met, and conduct continuing review of long-term research projects. Unless you are performing bench research, your project will require review of the research plan by the IRB. Research that includes the use of rDNA, biologicals, chemicals, or animals will be reviewed by other committees such as the institutional biosafety committee (IBC) or institutional animal care and use committee (IACUC). Your submission to the IRB generally has one of three outcomes: exemption, expedited review, or full committee review. Once your submission has been reviewed by the appropriate board, you will receive a letter of approval signifying that your research has met all the standards required for beginning your study.

Research Training

To submit an IRB application, investigators will need to show proof of research training or of meeting initial education requirements. This can include courses or modules on the Health Insurance Portability and Accountability Act (HIPAA) and ethics or informed consent training through the Collaborative Institutional Training Initiative (CITI) or National Institutes of Health (NIH). Requirements will vary by institution, so check with your mentor, preceptor, or director as to what requirements you will need to satisfy to have your application processed.

Submitting an Application

It is very important to undergo research training and submit your application as early as possible. You cannot begin your research project until you have obtained approval from the appropriate review board. The review process can be long, taking anywhere from 4 to 6 weeks to up to 3 to 4 months. And your application may not be approved as initially submitted. Do not worry if this happens. You may be asked to provide additional information or to modify collection tools, surveys, or letters of consent before approval can be obtained. Review the requirements for the application as you begin developing your research proposal so that you are aware early on of all that is involved. Be sure to submit all required information with your first application to ensure that the process is smooth and to prevent delays.

IRB Approvals

Obtaining approval from the IRB is a crucial step in the research process and provides legal protection to researchers. The approval letter signifies that the research plan has been deemed safe by a committee of experts. Also, if you are planning to publish your research down the road, pharmacy and medical journals will require you to include in the manuscript details on what type of approval was obtained and where. If you have obtained funding, granting agencies may not release funds until you have IRB approval.

IRB approvals typically expire after 1 year. After that, if you are still conducting the study you will need to apply for an extension or re-review of the application. There may also be cases in which you will need to notify the board of updates in your research as they occur (i.e., adverse effects, changes in protocol, changes to informed consent documents, questionnaires, other recruitment materials).

Developing a Curriculum Vitae

As part of the application process, you will need to submit a curriculum vitae (CV), either full or abbreviated, to the research board. In some cases the board will ask for only the principal investigator's CV, and in other cases all investigators involved must submit their CVs. As a student performing research, you may not yet have developed a CV. A resource that can help you with this is available at http://www.pharmacylibrary.com/resource/21. Your research mentor, research coordinator, or director can also provide you with guidance as you develop your CV. If you are a pharmacy resident or new practitioner, you will already have a CV developed; be sure to refine and update it regularly so you are prepared not only for this research requirement but also for seeking employment in the future. Obtaining feedback from co-residents, co-workers, residency directors, and research program coordinators will be helpful in refining your CV.

Additional Resource

1. Reinders TP. *The Pharmacy Professional's Guide to Résumés, CVs, & Interviewing*. 3rd ed. Washington, DC: American Pharmacists Association; 2011.

Approvals Checklist

☐ Undergo human subjects/informed consent/ethics training

☐ Submit an application to the appropriate research board (IRB, IBC, or IACUC)

☐ Develop (or refine) your curriculum vitae

CHAPTER 4

How Do I Collect, Organize, and Analyze Data?

Learning Objectives

1. Evaluate your research and determine what type of data collection tool it is necessary to create for your project.
2. Use the developed data collection tool to collect and organize your data.
3. Code and input your data into the statistical software you will be using.
4. Determine which statistical tests would be appropriate to use in your study.
5. Analyze your data.

Key Terms

- Data collection tool
- Coding data
- Inputting data
- Statistical tests
- Statistical software

He who sees things grow from the beginning
will have the best view of them.

—*Aristotle*

Now that you have designed your study, step 3 of the research process is collecting the data. An easy way to begin is to develop a data collection sheet or tool. The data collection tool will include the information about your study participants that you need to collect to answer your research question.

If we revisit our diabetes example, let's first think about the characteristics of our sample populations. The subjects should have diabetes, be obese, and use Lantus. Now, we need to think about how to further define those categories. What type of diabetes do the patients have? How is obesity defined? What other medications is the patient taking? Thus, type of diabetes, body mass index (BMI), and medications will become categories in the tool you use to collect information. What other considerations do you have? Demographic information such as age, race, and gender; duration of diabetes; severity of obesity; duration of Lantus use; and diet and exercise habits will need to be taken into account to provide a basis for comparing the groups and drawing conclusions in your study, so you should collect this information as well. Outcome measures also need to be included. Patient data on fasting blood glucose, 2-hour postprandial glucose (how often the subjects check their postprandial glucose and after which meal—breakfast, lunch, or dinner), and A1c should be obtained for your analysis. The conclusions you draw should be based on the inclusion and exclusion criteria you set for your study: that both populations must check their blood glucose levels at least twice a day and not be renally impaired. Thus, each subject needs to have a minimum of two daily glucose values and a creatinine clearance value. What is the time frame in which you are going to collect the data? The past year? The past 2 years? You will need to have a defined time period for your study. It is always best to collect as much information as possible; that way, when it comes to analysis, you will have a rich data set to look at and draw conclusions from.

Patient Recruitment

The inclusion and exclusion criteria you set for your research define your study patient population. You now need to think about how the subjects will be identified in your study. This can be done retrospectively or prospectively. Usually, student or resident research projects are retrospective, as time frames for performing the study are not long enough to ensure that an adequate sample size can be obtained if the data are collected prospectively. Data for retrospective chart reviews can be generated from the electronic medical record, clinic charts or schedules, admission or discharge reports, or prescribing reports.

Data for prospective studies would involve obtaining consent of the participant and active recruitment through letters or direct advertising (e.g., newspaper, radio, television, bulletin boards, Internet). Time for prospective patient enrollment would need to be accounted for in the research timeline, and this can take longer than anticipated.

Your study needs to contain an optimal sample size to ensure adequate power to detect statistical differences. Your research mentor or statistician can help you determine what this should be for your particular research project. There are also sample size and power calculators available online that can be useful. Try using one in preparation for meeting with your research mentor or statistician, and discuss with your co-investigators what you've found.

Using Data Collection Tools

Depending on where you are employed, where you are practicing as a resident, or whom you are working under as a student, you or your mentor or preceptor may be able to access data and run clinic reports that you can collect and input. If you are in a setting that does not use electronic medical records, you will need to manually review charts and collect the data. Find out what options are available to you.

In our current example, we are obtaining data through retrospective chart review. All of the collected data would be input into a spreadsheet or database. Each row of the spreadsheet would represent a subject (or case) within the study, and each column would represent the data (i.e., variable) being collected. For example, Column A would be Age, Column B would be Gender, and so on; there would be one variable per column. To satisfy IRB and HIPAA requirements, you should not collect any identifying information known as protected health information (i.e., name, birth date, address, social security number).

What if the study is survey based? How are things different? Actually, things are not that much different. The difference lies in the method by which you are collecting your study data. For example, with surveys, there are various methods for collecting information—electronically, by regular mail (paper survey), by telephone, or by interview. If you will be using an electronic survey, results can be downloaded into a database, eliminating data entry and associated errors—similar to running reports from an electronic database. Paper and telephone surveys or interviews will require manual collection and entry into a database.

Coding and Inputting Data

When inputting data into a database, data should be reported numerically and be consistent in format. It is best to keep variable names short so that you can view the entire spreadsheet at a glance; this decreases data-entry errors. For manual input of data from a survey, a codebook should be developed that defines the rules for how data entry will occur. You would develop a numeric code for each variable, list the code in the codebook, and share the codebook with any investigators who will be entering data so they can input it accordingly.

Creating a codebook is a way to help you stay organized and decrease errors. Your codebook is specific to your research only; it describes each variable and specifies how collected information will be entered into the database by you or other investigators. A sample survey, codebook, and accompanying spreadsheet are provided in Appendix G.

Cleaning Data and Maintaining Confidentiality

The process of data cleaning involves correcting any errors that might have occurred in the data file after the input stage. Typographical errors, extra spaces, and duplicate entries are common types of errors. Always go back to the survey where the discrepancy occurred to troubleshoot and correct errors.

It is important to remember that any research data and associated records need to be properly secured. If the data are paper based, they should be safely stored in locked cabinets in a secure room. If the data are electronic, create computerized data files that are secured with password protection.

Analyzing Data

Step 4 of the research process is analyzing data. Data are commonly organized and entered initially into a database such as Microsoft Excel or Microsoft Access. The data are then imported into statistical software programs for analysis (i.e., SPSS [IBM] or SAS [SAS Institute Inc.]). The statistical tests that are used depend on the types of variables and data you are collecting. Your mentor or statistician can guide you in using SPSS or SAS if you've never used the software before. If you would like to get familiar with SPSS, tutorials and free trials are available online.[1] Various resources are also available that can help you determine which tests would be most appropriate.

Reference and Additional Resources

1. IBM SPSS software. http://www-01.ibm.com/software/analytics/spss/. Accessed June 9, 2014.
2. Dawson-Saunders B, Trapp RG. *Basic & Clinical Biostatistics.* 4th ed. New York: McGraw-Hill; 2004. The primary focus is on statistics, including mathematical calculations and clinical applications.
3. Malone PM, Kier KL, Stanovich JE. *Drug Information: A Guide for Pharmacists.* 4th ed. New York: McGraw-Hill; 2012.
4. Iverson C, Christiansen S, Flanagin A, et al. *AMA Manual of Style: A Guide for Authors and Editors.* 10th ed. New York: Oxford University Press; 2007.

Collecting and Analyzing Checklist

☐ Create a data collection tool

☐ Develop a survey (as necessary)

☐ Code, input, and clean data

☐ Ensure that all research data are safely secured

☐ Analyze data

CHAPTER 5

How Do I Disseminate My Work?

Learning Objectives

1. Appropriately summarize the findings of your research.
2. Describe how to develop a descriptive title and concise abstract.
3. Design a research poster and presentation.
4. Develop the components of a research manuscript.

Key Terms

- Title
- Abstract
- Research posters
- Poster presentation
- Research manuscript
- Results
- Discussion
- Conclusions
- Acknowledgments
- References

Hofstadter's Law: It always takes longer than you expect,
even when you take into account Hofstadter's Law.
—Douglas Hofstadter

The final step of the research process involves reporting your findings. You have already begun formulating sections of your project by developing a research proposal; now it is time to refine those beginning sections and add the additional sections of Results, Discussion, and Conclusions.

Title and Abstract

Let's talk about titles and abstracts first. The title and abstract of your research project are very important. They are the first impression you give of your research, and people make a snap judgment within seconds as to whether they want to read more about your research. So it is extremely important to create a title and abstract that are clear, accurate, and concise and will grab and hold the reader's attention. Your goal is to make the reader stop and delve further into your research.

First, the title. As an example, let's see what we can do to improve the following title: "Establishing an Immunization Clinic." This title is not very descriptive. Where is the clinic being established? Who's managing the clinic? What kind of immunizations? Do not make your readers guess. If it takes too much work to understand the title, how likely is anyone to want to read more? Highly unlikely! Be clear and descriptive. A better title would be "Establishing a Pharmacist-Managed Meningitis Clinic in the Community Setting."

The abstract is a brief summary of the study, concept, or method described in the research manuscript. It introduces the reader to the objectives, methods, results, and conclusions of your report. Again, your goal is to make the reader want to read your full manuscript, so make a good impression. Ask yourself, Are the objectives clearly stated? Is the description of methods and materials understandable? Are the statistical tests used adequately described? Are the results presented in sufficient detail to support the conclusion? Is a sound conclusion being made? Is it clearly presented? Are there any practical implications of the information?

Abstracts are usually limited to 200–300 words, but the length is specified by the conference at which you may want to present your work or the journal in which you may want to publish it. Your mentor might like you to have experience presenting a poster and may have in mind a specific professional meeting or conference. Discuss this with your mentor, and create an abstract according to the meeting guidelines. Similarly, residency or capstone research programs may have specifications for abstract length; discuss this with your residency director or research program coordinator.

Why should you write an abstract? It may be required by the school or residency program. Even if you are not required to write an abstract, taking the time to write one and submit it to a professional organization for poster presentation will give you the opportunity to present your research in a peer-reviewed format. Writing an abstract is the initial step in submission of your work—to be accepted or rejected—for poster (or platform) presentation, and it is a necessary component of publishing manuscripts. Presenting your research at conferences and publishing it in journals are great ways to get involved in the profession—and to strengthen your CV. For a sample abstract, see Appendix H.

Research Posters

Research posters are a visual communication tool that summarizes the study, concept, or method. Why would you want to create and present a research poster? There are many benefits to you as a budding or even an experienced researcher. An effective poster helps you engage colleagues in the discovery of knowledge. Not only does it give you skills in developing an effective visual representation that summarizes your work, but it advertises your work to others as well. Presenting at local, state, and national conferences provides a platform for you to highlight your research and allows you to contribute to the profession through your research and scholarship. Discussing your research with those attending the poster session can also lead to potential research collaborations in the future.

The sections to include in a poster are Introduction/Background, Objectives, Methods, Results, Implications and Limitations, Conclusions, Acknowledgments/Disclosures, and References. The main difference between a poster and a manuscript is that the poster is more concise and elements of the poster (mainly the results) are represented in a visual rather than written manner. Sample posters using various designs are included in Appendix I.

Research Poster Tips

When developing the poster, you need to keep in mind the size, font, space, content, and visual elements (e.g., graphs, charts, tables). Posters are typically developed in Microsoft PowerPoint, with dimensions of 24 inches high by 48 inches wide. You can select this size by clicking on the PowerPoint Page Setup button under the Design tab.

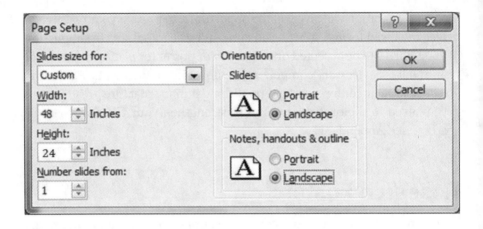

The font sizes should be a minimum of 32, and the styles should be basic, clean, simple, and easy to read. Some good font choices are Times New Roman, Arial, Calibri, and Verdana. The idea is to use a font that can be easily read up close and from afar. Posters should strike a good balance between content and visuals; to be visually appealing, they should appear symmetrical and uncrowded. Using bulleted statements tends to be easier on the eyes of the reader, as well as easier for the presenter to follow. Using bullets to highlight the most important points is more effective than developing sections in paragraph format. Graphs and charts for your poster can be made in Microsoft Excel or PowerPoint. Excel has various functions, so give yourself time to create and play with the graphs or charts and make them as visually appealing as possible. Add titles, data labels, and axis labels to make your graphs easy to read and interpret for both you and the audience members. Once your graph is completed, you can cut and paste it from Excel into your PowerPoint poster template. Alternatively, you can create charts or graphs in PowerPoint and cut and paste them directly into the template.

In creating the content of your poster, do not write in the first person. Your writing should be formal and scientific, similar to the research proposal. It should be clear and concise. After formulating each section, ask yourself, Would this description give the reader enough information about what was done? Tables, charts, and figures should be used when appropriate. The poster design should be kept standard and traditional; do not use colors or fonts that would distract the audience and ultimately take away from your message.

Once your poster is designed and you are ready to print, you can go to the website www.makesigns.com. Most posters are printed in glossy or matte finishes, sized at 36 by 72 inches, since conference poster boards generally accommodate posters the size of 4 feet by 8 feet. The conference you will be attending will have specific requirements for your presentation. For example, some conferences want you to include an icon of the professional organization on your poster, and they provide it for you to use when they accept the poster abstract. Be sure your poster follows the specifications for that conference. National professional organizations that accept student and resident poster submissions include the American Association of Colleges of Pharmacy (AACP), American College of Clinical Pharmacy (ACCP), American Pharmacists Association (APhA), and American Society of Health-System Pharmacists (ASHP). Discuss with your mentor which conference would be most suitable for submitting your research. Your mentor may also want you to consider local organizations. Once a conference has been chosen, go to the organization's website and find out when submissions are accepted and when the conference occurs; work this into your overall timeline for the year so that you have adequate preparation time.

Poster Presentations

Essentially, a research poster is a hybrid of a published paper and an oral presentation. During a poster presentation, you are orally presenting all of the sections that are included in a manuscript. Often, your school, residency institution, or workplace will have a recommended poster template for you to use. Find out if one is available or if you will need to create one. A sample poster template is provided in Appendix J.

After you've created your poster, you can then begin to work on the presentation. The presenter provides a short oral summary of the project for those visiting the poster session. The presentation is informal. It involves greeting the passerby, providing an overview of the research, and answering questions that the passerby has. Comments from the passersby can be addressed in the manuscript or used to enhance future work.

Poster Session Tips

Always arrive early for your poster session to locate where your poster should be set up. Find out if you need to bring your own pushpins or if the conference will be providing them. Expect to be available for the entire time allotted to your session. Try to greet and engage everyone who stops by to view your poster, and use the feedback you receive to strengthen your research manuscript. Do not become so engaged with one person that all others with questions or comments are ignored. A nice touch is to have available for distribution a page-sized printout of the full poster or a business card with contact information. Alternatively, you could include a section in your poster that says "For more information, contact," with your name and email address. This information would thus be contained in the page-sized printout. Approximately 20 copies should be enough to keep on hand and distribute.

Research Manuscripts

Let's revisit the research proposal that was discussed in Chapter 2 and Appendix D. As stated previously, components of the Introduction are a review of background literature, the rationale for and significance of conducting your research, and the purpose and objectives of your study. The Methods section describes your study design and how you conducted your study (e.g., associated procedures and protocols, endpoints) and explains your data collection and the statistical methods you used for analysis.

The manuscript sections that were not covered in Chapter 2 were the Results, Discussion, Conclusions, Acknowledgments, and Tables/Figures. Here, we will discuss these in depth. You should begin to incorporate these sections into your proposal after your data have been collected and analyzed. Once you've done this, your research proposal has become your research manuscript.

Results

For the Results section, I recommend that you begin backwards. In other words, create your tables and figures before you attempt to write your Results section. Your first table (or figure) should summarize the demographics or baseline characteristics of your study population. Subsequent tables should be created to address each objective of your study. Develop a concise but descriptive title for each table and figure. Always include N's at the end of the title. Table information should include the N's and percentages side by side. If you need to clarify or add any information, include this in footnotes at the bottom of the table or figure. Each journal may have a slightly different symbol or lettering sequence for footnotes, so be sure to review the journal's table and figure guidelines.

By creating the tables and figures first, you can ensure that your written description of the results is not an exact replica of what is represented in the tables or figures. The Results section should provide a summary (rather than a play-by-play) of what you found and should then refer the reader to the tables and figures you have created for further detail. Also note that this section should present your results but should save any discussion of the results for the Discussion section. Be accurate and clear in your writing.

Discussion

The Discussion section is composed of various parts. It is the only section in the manuscript in which authors have a "voice." Here, authors can provide their subjective thoughts and insights on the research performed, based on their previous experience and on common knowledge or expert opinion.

In this section, you can interpret your data and draw conclusions about your research question or hypothesis. Here you are able to provide answers to questions posed in the Introduction and to compare and contrast your findings with those available in the literature. How does your research compare to the existing literature?

Limitations of the research are also covered in the Discussion section. You are probably thinking, Why would I want to emphasize the flaws of my study? This is actually a very beneficial component of your analysis. It allows you as the author to consider the overall validity of the study. If authors realize the study limitations, they can consider those limitations in making conclusions. Thus, recognizing and stating limitations strengthens the impact of the work. What was your research unable to address? How could methods have been altered to provide more definitive results? Have potential problems or biases been identified that make the study inaccurate?

Another component of the Discussion section is implications: What is the impact of your research? To which populations would the study findings apply? How generalizable are the findings? What do the results mean to health care and to society? Do the findings suggest changes that need to be made in practice? It may be that current practice is supported by your data and results, in which case your recommendation may be to continue with current best practices. What future studies can be done to address this topic? What additional questions need to be asked and answered?

Take the time to think critically in evaluating and reflecting on your research. It is important that the conclusions you draw and the limitations and implications you identify are clearly supported by your study. Typically, no page length is specified for the Discussion section. You can write as much as you need to in order to address all of the points mentioned previously. The tone of the section should be formal and matter-of-fact.

Conclusions

How is the Conclusions section different from the Discussion? In this section, the author states major findings of the study. This section is much shorter than the Discussion section and is usually not much longer than a paragraph. Appendix K includes a sample research manuscript template for you to follow.

Acknowledgments

The acknowledgments section of the manuscript allows you to thank anyone who helped you with your research (but not co-authors on the project). For example, this could be someone who helped you with data collection, or maybe a statistician who helped with analysis. Consider whether you would like to acknowledge anyone in this section.

References

The reference section allows readers to locate the sources of your research. It also gives appropriate credit to the authors of your sources. Chapter 2 explained ways in which to collect and save reference information. Compile the references you have used throughout your research project, and organize them in the preferred style for the journal to which you plan to submit your manuscript.

Dissemination Checklist

☐ Develop a descriptive title and a concise abstract of your research project

☐ Submit your abstract to professional organizations for conference presentation

☐ Create a poster and prepare an informal presentation of your research (upon abstract acceptance)

☐ Print your research poster

☐ Begin writing the final sections (Results, Discussion, Conclusions, Tables/Figures, Acknowledgments, and References) of a research manuscript

CHAPTER 6

What's Involved in Publishing?

Learning Objectives

1. Describe internal and external peer-review processes.
2. Identify scientific pharmaceutical and medical journals to submit to.
3. Generate a research manuscript according to author guidelines.
4. Prepare a manuscript for online submission to a journal.
5. Outline a section in your curriculum vitae for research publications and presentations.

Key Terms

- Internal peer review
- External peer review
- Scientific journals
- Author guidelines
- Curriculum vitae—research experience

> *I believe in intuition and inspiration. Imagination is more important than knowledge. For knowledge is limited, whereas imagination embraces the entire world, stimulating progress, giving birth to evolution. It is, strictly speaking, a real factor in scientific research.*
>
> *—Albert Einstein*

Publishing a research manuscript is the final step in the research process. Not only is it a significant accomplishment, but it is a huge source of satisfaction—a living testament to the work you have completed. A published manuscript not only documents your contribution to the research literature but also allows you to disseminate information to a broad audience. Think of it as a way to make a lasting, meaningful contribution to the profession of pharmacy. In addition, it allows you to perpetuate the research cycle; it opens the way for others to continue to create new knowledge to solve existing or emerging challenges.

Internal Peer Review

After you've finalized your manuscript, you'll want to ask your mentor and those associated with your project to read it and provide feedback (if you haven't already been doing this along the way). After that, ask people who are not associated with your research to give you feedback. In essence, what you are doing is soliciting your own internal peer review. This helps ensure that your work is clear and understandable to those who are not involved in the project. You want your manuscript to be the best of the best when you are ready to submit it, with the goal of having it accepted by the journal of your choice. Consider any feedback you receive as one more tool for strengthening your manuscript and preparing it for publication. Make it a priority to carefully revise the manuscript to incorporate feedback, and discuss concerns with your reviewer. You may not agree with all of the suggestions you receive, but take note of any substantive changes and comments and address them.

Selecting Journals

How do you know which journal to submit to? Your mentor will be very helpful in guiding you to the most appropriate journal for your manuscript. How do you know which journals are available? A simple way to determine this is to search the PubMed database (www.pubmed.gov). Click on "Journals in NCBI Databases." From there, you can enter the topic of your research, and the database will generate titles of journals that may be applicable. You can also do research on your own regarding journals you think would be applicable. Go to those journals' websites and peruse the journal's aims and scope. Review the author guidelines; there you will find further information on the types of articles the journal publishes (e.g., commentary, original research, letters, review articles), and this will help you determine whether your work would be a good complement to the journal and its audience members. Have a discussion with your mentor about your findings. You want to have a Plan B in place in case Plan A does not work out. And if Plan A does not work out, don't be discouraged! Keep on trying, and you will achieve your goal of publication. It may take longer than you anticipated, but it will happen if you stay committed.

External Peer Review

Once you've submitted your manuscript to a journal, the editors will assign your manuscript to three to six reviewers around the United States who have experience with your research topic. The reviewers will evaluate your manuscript and provide feedback. This process usually takes 4 to 8 weeks. The reviewers will also make recommendations as to whether the manuscript is suitable for publication in that particular journal. Typical recommendations of the reviewers are accept, accept with minor revision, reject with reconsideration after major revision, or reject. The journal editors will take the reviewers' comments and final recommendations into account when they make their final decision.

Whether your manuscript is accepted or rejected, the editor will correspond with you to provide the reviewers' evaluations as well as their own. If the editors recommend rejection, use the reviewers' feedback to revise and strengthen your manuscript. Then move on to Plan B: Choose the next journal you thought was appropriate, format your manuscript to its specifications, and submit it again. Don't give up!

Manuscript Format and Layout

I cannot stress how important it is to follow your chosen journal's author guidelines. Ensure that you address all areas, from cover letters to title pages and correspondence information, manuscript formatting, referencing, table and chart construction, and footnotes. Journals usually provide a manuscript checklist for you to follow to ensure that all components are addressed; use this to keep you on track. The journal may require further paperwork such as conflict of interest forms or disclosure forms upon acceptance of your manuscript. Be aware of the requirements and procedures necessary to make the process smooth for you and all those involved.

Research Experience on Your CV

Once your manuscript is accepted, you can create a Publications section in your CV and include the citation there. Similarly, you can include a Presentations section for information on your poster or platform presentations. Having these in your CV sets you apart from others. Be proud, and strive to add even more to these sections in the future.

Publication Checklist

☐ Finalize your research manuscript

☐ Have various people internally peer review your work

☐ Select an appropriate journal to submit to

☐ Format your manuscript according to author guidelines provided by that journal

☐ Submit your manuscript via online submission to the journal

☐ Address correspondence from external reviewers and the editors thoroughly

☐ Develop (or refine) the Publication and Presentation sections of your CV

CHAPTER 7

Where Can I Go from Here?

Learning Objectives

1. Evaluate your research goals for the future.
2. Apply time management, organizational, and interpersonal skills to developing and completing future research projects.

Key Terms

- Keys to success
- Time management
- Collaboration

Keys to a Successful Career in Pharmacy Research

To be successful in conducting research in pharmacy, you have to remain dedicated. During your first year of research, you will lack experience and have a steep learning curve, with both successes and challenges along the way. As you continue to learn and gain experience, the successes and challenges will keep coming (research or otherwise), but you will be better able to address them. How you address the challenges will make all the difference.

Time, motivation, and perseverance play significant roles in how you perform and complete your research and achieve your goals. Re-evaluate your research goals at the end of the year, and determine your goals for the year ahead.

Collaboration

Collaborating with others makes it much easier to perform research. Stay connected with your research mentor, preceptors, professors, and colleagues. There may be a project on which you want to collaborate with them in the future. Since you've worked together before, you will be accustomed to their expectations, and you can expand your mentor–mentee relationship into a collaborative, collegial one.

Research Initiatives

Often, the easiest topic to select for your research is what you are already doing. Do not feel as though you have to go searching for the most novel idea or the latest and greatest breakthrough. No matter what practice setting you find yourself in after graduation, you can apply your research skills there. Performing research in your current practice area will showcase your expertise. You may want to work interprofessionally, helping to show the impact of services provided by a team of health professionals. Or you may want to get involved in local or state initiatives. Always be open to new prospects, and do not be afraid to take on unfamiliar things. When it comes to research, the sky's the limit.

Pharmacy Research Success Checklist

- ☐ Continue to develop and hone your research skills
- ☐ Keep in touch with your research mentor, professors, and preceptors
- ☐ Determine what your research goals are for the future
- ☐ Begin a new research project in collaboration with others

CHAPTER 8

Personal Stories from Pharmacy Research Mentors

Learning Objectives (for Chapters 8 through 10)

1. Describe mentor perspectives on personal research experiences.
2. Describe mentee perspectives on personal research experiences.
3. Reflect on and apply mentoring perspectives to your own research experiences.

Key Terms (Chapters 8 through 10)

- Mentors
- Mentees
- Self-reflection

A Clinical Pharmacist's Experience as a Research Mentor

Melissa Badowski, PharmD, BCPS, AAHIVP
Clinical Assistant Professor, Section of Infectious Diseases Pharmacotherapy

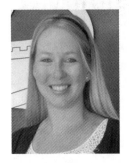

I never thought I would be excited about performing research as a clinical pharmacist. As a pharmacy student and resident, I looked at my preceptors in amazement and wondered how they could identify so many brilliant research ideas. Never did I imagine that I would become a mentor helping to engage others in the research process.

Initially, I was intimidated by the idea of research, but the patience and guidance of my research mentors helped me overcome my intimidation. They guided me through the fundamentals and gave me confidence that I could initiate and perform research.

As I started new clinical pharmacy services, I found many unanswered questions to investigate. By the end of a year I had at least 10 research ideas and wondered how I could pursue all of them. I began receiving correspondence from pharmacy students interested in research opportunities. When I contacted them, the students always said I was the only research mentor who had responded to their inquiries. These students were motivated to seek out research opportunities, so why shouldn't I expose them to research in clinical pharmacy?

I soon realized that many of the students did not know what research entailed. When I had explained the whole process and asked if they thought they could handle it, most were still up for the challenge. I interviewed my mentees—and they interviewed me. I wanted to be sure that I would help them achieve their goals and that they would help me achieve mine.

The characteristics I require of students, residents, and fellows performing research with me are accountability, open communication, attention to detail, and adequate time management. To assess whether they are truly interested in research, I assign them to undergo HIPAA and CITI training and to perform a literature search. If they do not complete these tasks in a timely fashion, that indicates to me that they are not truly committed to the research process, and I decline to initiate research with them.

I believe that supporting the mentee throughout the research process is essential, but I make sure not to micromanage. I state my expectations clearly and leave room for open communication and questions. Each week, I either meet with my mentees or correspond with them by email to be sure they are making adequate progress and to address any questions or concerns. Student research tends to be one semester long, while resident and fellow research is typically a year long. Most research involves individual projects, but in some cases when students are early in their pharmacy studies, I pair the student with a resident or fellow who can provide advice and experience from a different perspective. This also allows the resident or fellow to gain mentorship experience. All of the research performed by students, residents, and fellows is published as poster presentations.

I owe it to my mentees to provide them with an experience that ignites their passion for research. Most of the students and residents I mentor are engaging in research for the first time. If I fail to make a good impression, they will be turned off by research forever. It is important to make them feel that they are an active part of the research team. I encourage them to design the study, identify inclusion and exclusion criteria, create a database for data collection, submit paperwork for the IRB, and engage in the publication process.

My mentees have found that I am very enthusiastic about teaching the research process. I tell them that this is easy, since I am passionate about research. When my students and residents ask how I come up with research ideas, I tell them I was once in their position. I use my clinical practice site to my advantage. Where there are data lacking, there is a research opportunity.

Most of the research I perform with students and residents goes smoothly, but there are always areas for improvement. I have learned that I must be explicit in my directions and goals. When students and residents agree to do research, we devise a timeline to complete necessary steps, taking into consideration their coursework or rotation schedule. I have found that a timeline helps hold my mentees accountable. When collecting data, we go through the first few patient charts together and enter the data in the database. This helps ensure consistent data collection. I review their data in blocks based on the size of their study. With communication on at least a weekly basis, the lines of communication are open. I want my mentees to see me as approachable and committed to their learning throughout the research process. I always allow additional time for research if unforeseen issues arise. I do not want the research process to be filled with anxiety. I look at these mentor–mentee relationships as groundwork for future collaboration, and I want my mentees to feel equipped and confident to engage in research and to become mentors themselves.

It is very gratifying to see my mentees accomplish their goals, whether the goal be successful completion of a research project, publication, poster presentation, residency, or employment. I continue to accept research students and residents and look forward to showing them that research can be a positive and rewarding experience.

A Residency Research Director's Guide to Conducting Research

Vicki Groo, PharmD
Residency Research Director

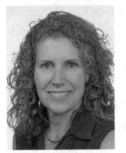

For pharmacy residents, working on a research project when they have multiple other responsibilities can be a time-management challenge. As an experienced residency research program director, I offer residents the following advice and insight on various steps in the research process.

Selecting a Project

Residency program preceptors and program directors often generate project ideas before the resident's arrival. In smaller programs, a project based on the needs of the institution may be assigned. Larger programs may compile a list of projects for residents to choose from. In the latter case, I encourage residents to discuss projects in detail with a potential mentor, to learn more about expectations and mentoring style and the fit with their needs and experience. For example, a resident with no research experience may need hands-on mentoring and will want a preceptor who is willing to provide that time and expertise. A less common scenario is a resident who comes to the program with a research project or question in mind. In this case, I would recommend that the resident discuss the idea with the residency program director, with the goal of identifying a mentor and assessing feasibility at the institution.

Developing the Protocol

Protocol development begins with a thorough literature search on the topic of interest. Sections of the protocol include Background/Purpose, Objectives/Hypothesis, and Methods (i.e., study population, inclusion/exclusion criteria, time period, data collection). A data collection form should be submitted with the protocol. The protocol should conclude with study limitations, risks, and benefits. Even though most residency projects are chart reviews, there is still a risk of loss of confidentiality. The protocol needs to describe a plan for minimizing this risk (e.g., stating how and where data will be stored and how identifiers will be protected).

Before finalizing a proposal for IRB review, residents often give a 10-minute presentation on the background and methods to an audience of faculty, clinicians, and students. This presentation serves two purposes: (1) the audience can assess whether the resident has a solid understanding of what the research entails and can provide constructive feedback and (2) the resident gets public speaking practice.

Obtaining IRB Approval

Navigating an institution's IRB can be intimidating, especially if the resident has not done this previously. Completing a project in a single year is challenging, so getting IRB approval as soon as possible is key to staying on track. Tips for getting approval are to be sure to have a well-written protocol, to have the correct paperwork filled out, and to use the correct language, especially in regard to risk, benefit, and confidentiality. I recommend that residents have a colleague with IRB experience review the protocol and IRB paperwork prior to submission, and that the resident submits it for IRB review no later than mid-September at the beginning of the residency.

Collecting Data

It doesn't matter how well a project is designed if the data are not managed in such a manner that the output can be analyzed. Residents often struggle with this because of a lack of experience. Residents should know what data management tools and programs are available to them. More important, they need to know what statistical program will be used to analyze the data. The statistical software and analysis plan will dictate how the database should be set up. The residency program may offer discussions on data management or reviews of statistics to help provide an overview. Ask your program director or residency coordinator about this.

The data collection is the most time-consuming part of completing a project. Do not wait until the last minute to do this. Chart reviews can become tedious, and they often take longer than expected. If the project is a chart review, the resident should set aside a certain number of hours per week for collecting data. It is easy to put this off when the resident has patient care duties, staffing duties, and other residency-related projects. The number of hours set aside should be based on how long it takes to collect data on one patient and how many patients are in the study. Enlisting other pharmacists working on the ward or clinic, students, and co-investigators as researchers on your project can also be helpful.

Analyzing Data

Often, the resident is relieved when data collection is finally done, thinking that analysis of the data will be a breeze. Analyzing data takes longer than you think. If Excel is used, data will need to be sorted and formulas added. If a statistical software program is used, data will need to be uploaded and labeled. If a statistician is involved, he or she may have many projects to work on at once, so the turnaround time may be longer than you expect.

When the data analysis is complete, it should be reviewed by a second set of eyes to be sure the results make sense and are valid. As a residency project mentor, I have come across many mistakes in this area. One of the biggest mistakes was when a resident sorted an Excel spreadsheet, completed the analysis, and had an abstract accepted for presentation at a major medical meeting, only to have to withdraw it later. It was discovered that the sort function was done incorrectly so that only the data from a particular column were sorted (rather than the whole dataset) and the data no longer matched up with the subject, and therefore the analysis was invalid. Typos in Excel can also create errors. When I was reviewing a dataset, the standard deviation on serum creatinine was quite large and just didn't look right. Inspecting the raw data, I found a couple of data points entered as 12.1 rather than 1.21 and 11.0 rather than 1.10.

Presentation of the Project

Residents can gain experience through poster presentations at professional meetings and oral research presentations at their regional residency conference in the spring. Before submitting final slides for a conference, residents should practice the presentation with an audience that can give constructive feedback in regard to overall presentation style, slides, content, and conclusions.

Writing a Manuscript

As the year is nearing a close and the residency conference presentation is over, staying motivated to finish a manuscript often becomes challenging. One way to overcome this challenge is to write the manuscript in sections.

Writing to get it done and quality writing are often two different papers. To improve the quality of writing, a good place to start is to seek constructive feedback from your mentor. Just as with your IRB submission, it is always a good idea to have another person review your work. Ideally, it would be someone who is not familiar with the project and brings a fresh set of eyes to see if your writing is clear.

Time Management

The project is something the resident needs to work on throughout the year, in contrast to rotations that change every month or a seminar or drug information monograph that is due on a specific date. With the many responsibilities of a resident, the research project can often fall by the wayside. Setting deadlines for completion of the various components is a great way to keep on track.

Project Quality

Mentors and residents should meet regularly to assess progress and discuss any concerns or issues with the project. Sometimes a project objective or design needs to be altered as a result of unexpected circumstances. A recent example at our institution was a prospective study on smoking cessation. It turned out that patients were declining participation because they did not want to be randomized to the usual care arm of the study. The study was then redesigned to use a historical control and a prospective intervention. If it had not been for the resident's good communication with the mentor about enrollment problems, the project would have been a failure.

The key to success is setting deadlines and having a fresh set of eyes to review the project. Particular attention should be given to the protocol methods, the IRB paperwork prior to submission, and the manuscript. Residents should also have a chance to practice presentations to a group unfamiliar with the project before presentation at a regional or national meeting.

Mentor–Mentee Relationships

Monsheel Sodhi, PhD
Assistant Professor, Pharmacy Practice

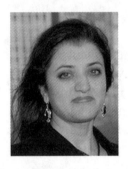

Mentorship is both a challenge and a joy in academia. I stand on the shoulders of my former mentors and try to emulate their best mentorship skills to benefit my mentees. I consider the success of the trainees under my mentorship as an important deliverable of my laboratory. I have heard that some peers are daunted by the upfront investment required for training temporary students, but I consider engaging bright, fresh minds to be a benefit to the laboratory because of the mentees' exuberance, their potential to assist once trained, and their potential to become bitten by the research bug and contribute to our research field in the longer term.

The degree of difficulty of academic research is surprising to students emerging from years of structured courses. During my doctoral studies, several peers and juniors sought my support. In those days I could provide only time, a positive attitude, and scientific suggestions. These interactions and my own experience as a mentee have provided useful insights that I can channel to help my current and future trainees. Initially I meet with prospective mentees in an informal interview to discover their goals, both long-term and short-term. If I see opportunities to help them succeed, I agree to be their mentor. If not, I often redirect them to a colleague who can help. Several very goal-directed mentees have passed through my laboratory. My task as a mentor is simpler when they know what they want, because I can try to help them achieve the goal they have defined.

Psychology students and graduates often gravitate to my laboratory because of our focus on psychiatry research. These individuals are often well organized, with good communication skills, and they are proactive about making progress in their careers. These students may have no knowledge of basic chemistry, which presents obstacles to understanding the biochemistry and genetics being studied in my research group. Although it is courageous to step into the unknown and take on the challenge of "wet-bench" training in molecular neuroscience, realistically there are obstacles to consider. The predictor of success here is whether the student has taken high school courses in chemistry at the very least. If so, then bringing the trainee up to speed with doctoral-level biochemistry is difficult but not impossible. If students have avoided chemistry throughout their academic career, then it is probable that they dislike the subject and find it difficult. Unless they are prepared to make a herculean effort to fill the gap in their knowledge base, they will be destined to never perform experiments beyond the level of a junior technician. This is because the foundation for understanding the experimental techniques we perform will be absent.

My recommendation now, after one difficult mentor–mentee relationship, is that these students need to study basic chemistry and biochemistry courses outside laboratory hours, preferably before starting a research project with my team. If family commitments preclude this extra effort, then I advise prospective mentees to seek out alternative training that will build on their strengths. As a mentor, it is my responsibility to prevent my mentees from struggling and becoming demoralized in the process. One gifted psychology major did in fact rise to the challenge and, although new to biochemistry, he acquired basic wet-bench skills and completed a short project in my laboratory to get a flavor of basic (nonclinical) research. He subsequently earned his MPhil in neuroscience at Oxford and won an award for his research with my support. He is now a faculty member in a department of psychology. Although there were potential difficulties, these were anticipated and overcome through the maturity, intellect, and drive of the mentee.

Another type of mentee is the clinician trainee who is attracted to my laboratory because of our focus on psychiatric disorders. Such potential mentees include residents in psychiatry, medicine, and pharmacy training programs. One psychiatry resident met with me for 2 hours twice monthly for his residency research project. This physician and I worked together for a year to generate publishable pharmacogenetic data. My mentee won two awards for presenting this research, became chief resident, and is currently working in a private clinical practice. I learned from this mentoring experience that despite their intellectual ability, trainees may be able to use this research experience only to boost their competitive advantage in a nonresearch-oriented job market. Nevertheless, this exceptional clinician will undoubtedly be better prepared than his colleagues when pharmacogenetics becomes more widely integrated into the clinical practice of psychiatry.

On occasion, clinicians underestimate the time required to perform research. Take, for example, an informal mentee who was working in a different laboratory. She was a medical doctor from Europe and considered her year of sponsored research to be a break so that she could start her family and experience living in the United States. This misconception was based on the lack of formal structure of research hours compared with the structure of a busy clinical schedule. In reality, students with just a year to complete a research project need to work incredibly long hours to learn new skills, master the concepts of research design, and collect data that are publishable. This student did not reach her full potential during that year. Nevertheless, she is continuing to contribute to clinical research after returning to Europe. I learned from this experience that detailed expectations must be stated clearly at the start of a mentor–mentee relationship.

The translational (clinical) focus of my laboratory is also attractive to graduate students in pharmacy and medical training programs. These students are some of the brightest that I have mentored. Biochemistry is not a prerequisite of many pharmacy courses, so I recommend extra reading for these students before they start their research projects. A medical student mentee who worked with me for a sponsored summer internship was excited by the research but daunted by the degree of difficulty it entailed. Although he was a pleasure to include in my team and displayed talent and potential, I had to advise this student to focus on performing well in the upcoming medical licensing exam rather than extending his research into the next semester. Another clinical student, in a foreign pharmacy program, learned English within 6 months with intensive didactic courses. He subsequently grasped concepts and laboratory techniques quickly and within the space of a few weeks has performed experiments with minimal supervision.

Undergraduate students are also a pleasure to mentor. These trainees are excited by the discoveries that are possible, and they are often aiming to apply for graduate school to become clinical practitioners or research scientists. My expectation is that at the very least, these bright minds contribute to the goals of my laboratory. At best, they may be infected by the challenge and excitement of research and perhaps contribute to scientific discovery later on in their careers. Although their initial goal is to gain research experience so that they can strengthen their applications to graduate school, they inadvertently become members of our laboratory family and are supported in many ways by my research team. This interaction provides a more personal environment for the students than they find in large undergraduate lecture halls.

These students clearly want to check off requirements for applying to graduate school, and they want to assist in my laboratory in addition to volunteering in other capacities (e.g., in clinical practice). These students may not have a passion for research, but they are highly motivated and conscientious. One such student followed instructions to the letter without taking notes, and her levels of attention and memory were impressive. She went on to win medals for being the top student in both the bachelors of neuroscience and bachelors of biology undergraduate courses. She is currently in medical training, which was her immovable goal. Another talented undergraduate student was assigned to my laboratory after successfully competing for a summer internship. He continued as a research assistant with me after graduating. This mentee integrated into my research team easily, and he was generally excited about life, his future, and science. His exuberance translated into a high level of achievement, including winning a research prize and co-authoring a book chapter with me. He received offers from a number of medical schools and is now studying medicine in his home state. These goal-directed mentees are a pleasure to work with.

Occasionally, mentorship is more challenging. Not all students remain certain of their goals, and in these cases success takes longer. A student mentee with strong intellectual, communication, and organizational skills habitually changed her mind about her career goals during the time she was in my laboratory. She had initially decided to pursue a career in scientific research and apply for graduate school. I worked with her for 12 months to design a project that would be of publishable quality and that she could present at the Society for Neuroscience meeting being held in her home state that year. The mentee wanted to return home to live, and employers and graduate programs in her home state would be well represented at that meeting. We surpassed expectations, and she won a travel award to present her work at the conference. Before the conference, however, she changed her mind about applying to a PhD program, but she persisted in collecting her prize and presenting at the conference to boost her resume. After some months of uncertainty, she found a position as a research technician in a neuroscience laboratory in her home state. Returning home reinvigorated her prior ambition to study medicine, and her applications to medical school will be boosted by a scientific publication we have in preparation. This experience taught me that my hopes for a mentee may not always align with the mentee's own goals.

So, mentorship can take unexpected directions. Establishing personal boundaries is essential to the development of a mutually respectful, mature mentor–mentee relationship. Regular meeting times and planned milestones are vital to the mentee's success. Mentorship is a two-way process requiring active participation of both mentor and mentee. The mentee must have goals, ambition, a strong work ethic, and the passion to learn. The mentor must be brave enough to risk giving true feedback so that the mentee can grow.

Mentorship is based on trust, and therefore feedback can be received in a beneficial manner only by someone who is mature, driven, and enthusiastic. Feedback requires an emotional investment on the part of the mentor. It is not pleasant to give negative feedback when it is needed, but it is a duty to help your mentee improve and succeed. Mentors also have a duty to delve into the depths of their own past failures and successes and give the mentee their most honest, considered advice. And most important, mentors should celebrate the successes of their mentees. I eagerly await news of the achievements of my mentees, past and present. I am sure that given the talent I am privileged to help nurture, these trainees will find novel ways to grow. It is a pleasure to see mentees extend the wings that start to develop during their training, to fly, succeed, and make us all proud.

CHAPTER 9

Personal Stories from Pharmacy Student Research Mentees

Research in My Second Year of Pharmacy School

Dalia J. Yousif, PharmD Candidate
Class of 2015

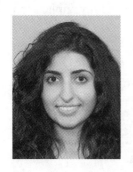

As a second-year pharmacy student I became involved in the specialty pharmacy service in an ambulatory care setting. This service had been established less than 2 years before my arrival, and it was rapidly expanding to meet the needs of patients receiving specialty drugs. The service was made successful by pharmacists who valued clinical skills, innovative ideas, and positive patient outcomes. As one of the many students affiliated with that specialty pharmacy, I was offered the opportunity to start my own research project. Because of my interests and career goals, my mentor recommended the topic of patient satisfaction. Over a year later, I completed a project titled "Patient satisfaction with health-system-based specialty pharmacy services compared with usual care."

I began my project with a literature search on patient satisfaction tools in various pharmacy settings. Specialty pharmacy was a relatively new and expanding field, and I found that no survey tools had been previously established to test patient satisfaction. I then performed a literature search on methods of writing and conducting surveys. I started with a 5-point questionnaire, which developed into a 27-question survey tool. I meticulously reviewed the survey wording, simplicity, grammar, and layout to ensure that the questions would be understood by all patients, regardless of their background. Selecting the questions for the survey was a challenge. The chosen questions covered service satisfaction and future opportunities.

After months of revision, I decided to administer the survey not only to patients at the specialty pharmacy but also to patients at competitor pharmacies. My research mentor, who managed the specialty pharmacy, was flexible and supported this new research design. She introduced me to the clinical pharmacist, who had experience creating survey tools and was able to help me improve my survey. I administered a pilot survey to 10 participants and quickly realized that some adjustments were still needed. I made the final revisions and increased the patient population to ensure that there would be enough consenting participants.

With my mentor and the clinical pharmacist as my co-authors, I was designated as the primary investigator in charge of getting IRB approval. I was excited by the opportunity and ready to work. Creating the IRB protocol and application required frequent revisions, especially since my co-authors had far more research experience than I did. As expected, I received feedback requiring me to adjust, clarify, and edit certain areas of my application before it could be approved.

After IRB approval, data collection could begin. As the sole person responsible for data collection, I needed to set aside enough time every week for the task, so I committed to 10 hours per week. After 4 weeks, I met with my co-authors for a midpoint evaluation of our research results. To our surprise, even with a small sample size of 50 participants, our results already showed that patients were far more satisfied with services from our health-system specialty pharmacy than with usual care.

With these preliminary results, I was asked to attend a staff meeting and present the findings to the pharmacy practice department. Then I completed my data collection with 100 patients, and I was fortunate to receive further support from the pharmacy practice department, which offered professional statistical analysis of the data. I recently submitted an abstract of my project for a poster presentation at an ASHP meeting, and I am awaiting statistical analysis so that I can begin writing a manuscript with my co-authors.

Doing research this past year has taught me many things. First, having a mentor who was knowledgeable and supportive has been the reason for my success and my passion in carrying out this study. Second, a practice environment that is innovative and tracks patient outcomes always offers students opportunities for research that fits their interests. The key to success is knowing that quality research requires time, patience, and flexibility. Revisions are to be expected! Finally, I learned that students' success is due in large part to their mentors, and I sincerely thank mine for their knowledge, guidance, and support.

How Research Changed My Career Outlook

Hyungsik Ahn, BS, PharmD Candidate
Class of 2015

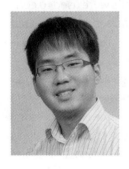

Although I had experience with research in my undergraduate years, I've found a whole new level of research experience in the professional degree program. During my first year of pharmacy school, I gained extensive experience in the areas of cancer and topoisomerase II-targeting drugs using yeast cells. Although I started pharmacy school thinking I would work in community practice, that goal changed because of my research. In my first semester I questioned faculty members and more advanced students to learn about the research being conducted on campus. Thus, I found out about a list of faculty conducting research and their current projects. The project that interested me was using topoisomerase II-targeting drugs on yeast cancerous cells, and I immediately contacted the faculty member in hopes of becoming involved in it.

Actually, I didn't have much choice in research projects. Since students do not learn the pathophysiology of cancer until our third year, I lacked the extensive background knowledge of cancer needed to support research on my topic of interest. Fortunately, the faculty member I contacted had a project in mind that he hoped to give someone to explore. I'd be lying if I did not acknowledge that I was afraid I might not be able to understand the project, but I was willing to go forward anyway.

As I began the project, my mentor had one of his postdoctoral research colleagues train me in all the procedures I would be using throughout the project. This researcher provided me with procedures and protocols that I would use and supervised me. She continued to oversee my work until I was comfortable carrying out the procedures by myself and able to reproduce the results that she would obtain if she carried out the procedures. Some of the procedures I learned were plasmid transformation, drug sensitivity analysis, and western blotting. Initially I struggled to finish these procedures alone, but after a month and a half of training and repetition, I was able to do the procedures from beginning to end without assistance. When I finished my first western blotting by myself, I was annoyed that it had taken so long for me to be able to do this successfully. But more important, it made me think about other projects in which I could apply my new skills and techniques.

The core of my project was transforming a new cell with a new vector through plasmid transformation and then using western blotting to confirm the successful transformation. The newly transformed cells were used to conduct a drug sensitivity analysis with topoisomerase II–targeting drugs such as etoposide. Drug sensitivity analysis was conducted by treating the transformed yeast colonies with different concentrations of the topoisomerase II-targeting drugs and calculating the survival percentage after incubation.

I was able to present the results of this project as a poster and as a short oral presentation at the college's annual research day. I had hoped to continue this research as a second-year pharmacy student, but my strict schedule as a second-year student didn't allow me to continue. My experience working in a pharmacy research laboratory caused me to think about continuing my education after the PharmD degree, as a PhD student.

There are only a few people with whom I have interacted who have amazed me with their knowledge and their passion for what they do, and my mentor was one of them. When I was having difficulty understanding the material and the logic behind the experiments, he motivated me and kept me from giving up. He helped me to not lose focus when I was struggling to produce results from the experiments—another time when I would have quit if not for my mentor's words. Without his help and encouragement, I would not have reignited my love for research and experienced what research is like in the pharmaceutical field.

After this exposure to research, I have decided to become a pharmacist researcher. I hope to find employment in the pharmaceutical industry and work in product development. I would like to carry out drug trials and develop new medications to improve patient care.

CHAPTER 10

Personal Stories from Pharmacy Resident Research Mentees

Learning the Ropes of Research: My Residency Research Experience

Laura Means, PharmD
PGY2 Critical Care Resident

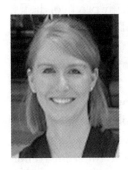

Research is a required component of residency training, and there is much to be gained from the experience. When they hear about research, pharmacy students typically envision PhDs in white coats working in a lab with chemicals. This is how I had envisioned research during my time as a student, but it could not be further from my experience as a postgraduate year 1 (PGY1) pharmacy practice resident. Instead, I had the opportunity to do clinical research that involved real patients and to find outcomes that could help make a difference in readmission rates.

At the beginning of the year, my residency class was presented with a list of possible research topics. My interest area was critical care, but since many other people shared that interest, I knew it would be difficult to get a critical care project. Therefore, I turned to infectious disease projects, as infectious diseases often affect critically ill patients. I have since realized that your research does not necessarily have to be in your specific area of interest, because the exercise of doing research, the effort put into the project, and the lessons learned are what will help you obtain the residency or job that you want. My mentor proposed retrospectively looking at patients discharged with outpatient parenteral antimicrobial therapy (OPAT) to assess the readmission rate and potential reasons for readmission. After discussing this idea with my mentor, I was intrigued by the possibility of finding a risk factor for readmission and potentially addressing that factor. I also knew it was important for me to have a mentor to support me through the process and be available for questions.

Initiating research can be daunting: deciding on the initial research idea as well as primary and secondary endpoints and then deciding on data collection points. Once you've done this, you should present the information to someone not involved in your research. I did this by giving a 15-minute presentation to a group of residents and faculty. This process helped assure my mentor and me that I hadn't overlooked things during development of the protocol. Outside faculty can also provide different suggestions for assessing the same endpoint or raise concerns about pitfalls not previously considered. After going through this process, I was able to refine my final data points and move on to the IRB application. Preparing and submitting the IRB application is a learning experience and takes many protocol drafts. My mentor and I exchanged at least a half dozen drafts of my protocol before finally submitting it to the IRB.

October 1, 2013, was a great day. My IRB submission had been accepted, and the real fun would begin. The goal was to enroll 200 subjects in my research, but I didn't know that would entail going through 592 medical records to assess them for study inclusion and then collecting 49 individual data points on each of the 216 subjects included. Actually, I admit that I enjoyed going through patients' charts and seeing the different trends emerge.

More exciting, and somewhat nerve-racking, was analyzing my data. I was eager to see if any factor was significantly more likely to lead to readmission of the patients receiving OPAT. Learning to use statistical software (SAS) to analyze the data took practice, as this program was completely foreign to me, but luckily I had a mentor who could use the program and teach me the basics. After compiling all the results, I was relieved to see that there were three independent predictors for readmission and that my research had not been in vain! With identified predictors for readmission, patients can be assessed more closely before being discharged with OPAT, with the goal of reducing readmission rates.

It is a huge relief to have analyzed all your data and have your results in hand. You must keep in mind, though, that there are still presentations to be made and a manuscript to generate. All residents in my program are required to present at the Great Lakes Pharmacy Resident Conference. A 20-minute presentation of your research and findings is given to an audience filled with residents from different programs, your mentor, your residency director, other residency directors, and faculty from other programs. The nice part about giving these presentations is that you know the data you collected better than anyone else does! My research has been presented to two infectious disease physicians involved in the project and then further shared with the anti-infective subcommittee of the hospital to discuss the potential impact on our patient population. I was also extremely fortunate to have my research accepted for oral presentation at the 2014 IDWeek meeting in Philadelphia, making all of the hard work even more satisfying.

Over the course of this research project, I've learned a great deal. It is important to pick a project that you are interested in, or the hours you put into it might seem more brutal than necessary. Pick a research mentor who will provide you with the type of guidance that you need, and discuss your needs with that person beforehand. Know that there will be many drafts of everything as your prepare your project. Be open to ideas and suggestions from outside faculty to improve your project. Once you've analyzed your data, be open to any opportunity that arises for you to present your research or publish your manuscript, because the more experience you get on this initial project, the more skills you will have for the next project you undertake. Although I do not plan on research being the only focus in my career, it will be a portion of it. I have acquired a variety of skills, and I look forward to my next research project as a PGY2 critical care pharmacy resident.

Research Strategies from a Resident's Perspective

Shubha Bhat, PharmD
PGY2 Ambulatory Care Resident

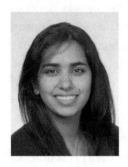

Residency, in a year, is designed to provide a well-rounded experience in areas ranging from patient care to practice management and research. Depending on a resident's background and future career goals, the research components required by a residency program can be an exciting or a daunting prospect. Use the following strategies to help optimize your research skills as a resident.

1. Before engaging in a research project, first do some research of your own.
    a. Identify what you hope to get out of your experience and where research fits into your career goals. In your future job, will you be expected to conduct quality improvement projects or publish manuscripts? Although it takes years of experience and education to become a top-notch researcher, creating an optimal research experience can provide you with a strong foundation—but it is important to set research goals first.
    b. Determine clinical areas of interest. A research project is designed to be long-term, so picking a topic that interests you makes the hours of data collection bearable. Also, this is a topic you will talk about extensively at resident research conferences and during interviews.
    c. As a newcomer to an institution, you may be provided with a list of research ideas; however, it is up to you to develop the project. Once you have accomplished steps a and b, set up meetings with mentors to determine whether their expectations align with your research goals. To ensure that the mentor is able to provide adequate research guidance and expertise, ask if he or she has worked with residents previously and what research projects have been completed at that institution. A

thriving mentor–mentee relationship is crucial to a successful residency research project, as you will be communicating with that mentor for the entire year. Furthermore, depending on your future goals, the mentor might assist with letters of recommendation or might be asked to comment on your research abilities.

2. Be aware of available resources.
   a. Depending on your institution, you may have access to certain tools such as SPSS or REDCap (from Vanderbilt Institute for Clinical and Translational Research) for data collection. Statisticians may be available through the department to assist with data analysis. Seminars or classes on research methods may be offered to augment your understanding. Use ASHP's new-practitioner comprehensive research resources center (http://www.ashp.org/menu/MemberCenter/SectionsForums/ NPF/Getting-Started) for additional tips. Reach out to your mentor to see what opportunities are available.
3. Once you start your research project, set deadlines.
   a. Each stage of a research project, from submitting an IRB application to collecting data to writing a manuscript and designing a poster, takes time, but in light of daily residency duties it is easy to delay these tasks until the deadline is close. Instead, designate time weekly to work on your research project. You will thank yourself for this in the end.

Finally, and perhaps this advice from Woody Allen is applicable to your entire residency, "If you're not failing every now and then, it is a sign you are not doing anything very innovative."

As a pharmacy student who participated in data collection and poster presentations, I found research to be exciting. By the middle of my PGY1 training, I had refined my career goals to include research responsibilities, and thus academia became an attractive prospect. Going into PGY2, I identified my research passion to be outcomes-related research, and from a list of projects provided I chose to investigate the outcomes of a pharmacist-managed heart failure medication titration clinic. I tailored my research goals to meet the job expectations of a faculty member, such as presenting posters at conferences and publishing manuscripts. My mentor graciously allowed me to design the project and provided endless feedback for refinement.

Identifying the optimal study design was a challenge, and I reached out to other faculty members and used the ASHP research resources center. Once I obtained IRB approval, I attended a seminar on how to use REDCap and created a data collection set. At first, data collection was cumbersome since I was not familiar with the institution's electronic medical record system, but after reviewing many patients' charts I found it easier. However, I wish I had done a better job of setting my own data collection deadlines. It would have been less burdensome to review at least 5–10 patient charts per day instead of 15–20 per day as the residency program's deadline for completion of data collection approached. My mentor assisted with data analysis, and I am now in the process of writing the manuscript, with the hope of publishing my findings in the next 6 months.

With each challenge I encountered, I gained a better understanding of research concepts, and I established a long-lasting relationship with my research mentor. I am now walking away with stronger research skills, which I will continue to use and refine in my new role as clinical assistant professor. Residency is an excellent career steppingstone, and I hope you will seize all the opportunities offered, especially in the area of research.

Mentoring Checklist

- [ ] Reflect on mentor and mentee perspectives on research
- [ ] Apply advice and insight to make your research experience a positive one
- [ ] Consider becoming a research mentor in the future

Afterword

They say that your experiences shape your outlook on life. I am so very grateful to the wonderful mentors I have had in research throughout my own pharmacy career. They never tired of explaining, training, and encouraging; their dedication and passion continue to be my inspiration in assisting future generations of pharmacists with their research efforts.

Every researcher must begin somewhere. And the research journey is not a simple one. It is full of twists and turns, with obstacles to be overcome and learning experiences to be had. Your first full research project will increase your skills and confidence in performing research tremendously. An open mind and a willingness to persevere are the keys to pharmacy research success. I guarantee it is a worthwhile endeavor. Best of luck to each of you!

Self-Reflection on Brainstorming a Research Idea

What type of research is most interesting to you? What research area or topic do you think you would like to get involved in? How do you think you can make a difference in this area? For yourself? For patients? For the profession? Take some time to reflect on these questions.

Potential Research Topics and Associated Research Questions

Research Area/ Discipline	Research Topic	Research Question
Clinical research	Asthma	What is the safety of long-acting beta agonists in children with asthma?
	Diabetes	Is there an association between vitamin B12 deficiency and metformin use in patients with type 2 diabetes?
	Hypertension	What is pharmacists' impact on attaining goal blood pressure in hypertensive patients in underserved areas?
	Infectious diseases	Is there a role for ceftaroline as an alternative to linezolid?
	Smoking cessation	How do outcomes in a veteran population with intensive phone management by pharmacists for tobacco cessation compare with standard care?

Research Area/ Discipline	Research Topic	Research Question
Laboratory research	Breast cancer	Are there new genes linked with an increase in breast cancer that can be discovered?
	Immunosuppression	What is the role of dendritic and T cells in immunosuppression?
	Meningitis	Can a new vaccine be developed to treat meningitis B?
	Neurotoxicology	Does acrylamide alter neurotransmitter-induced calcium responses in primary neurons of juvenile rats?
Educational research	Admissions	Do multiple mini-interviews (MMIs) provide a more successful approach than traditional interviews to admitting well-rounded students to colleges of pharmacy?
	Cultural competence	How do fourth-year pharmacy students self-assess cultural competency training during advanced pharmacy practice experiences?
	Didactic coursework	Can YouTube videos be used to enhance the student learning experience in a first-year physiology course?
	Research training	Does research training within a doctor of pharmacy program have an effect on practice as a pharmacist?

Successful Mentor–Mentee Relationships

Mentor Responsibilities	Mentee Responsibilities

1. Build the relationship.
  • Be approachable and flexible
  • Demonstrate sensitivity; listen thoughtfully and attentively as research interests and goals are discussed and shared by the mentee
	1. Listen.
	  • Question for clarification
	  • Establish goals and timelines

2. Establish protected time.
  • Meet with the mentee as often as agreed upon
	2. Be curious; be accountable.
	  • Be prepared for meetings; be flexible about meeting times

3. Be compassionate.
  • Enable but do not rescue
	3. Be open-minded; accept challenges.
	  • Gain the full measure of one's talents

4. Tacitly guide, advise, and nurture.
  • Maintain the mentee's confidence, and vice versa
	4. Accept constructive criticism.
	  • Move on; avoid self-pity

5. Encourage responsibility.
  • Provide timely feedback
  • Be committed to the success of the mentee
  • Empower the mentee
	5. Exercise accountability.
	  • Follow through
	  • Be aware of what is taking place
	  • Take initiative; plan work; pay attention to details

Mentor Responsibilities	Mentee Responsibilities

6. Teach about the research process.
  • Encourage successes, and trouble-shoot challenges together
	6. Recognize experience is a great teacher.
	  • Be open to learning from others' personal experiences
	  • Be reflective and gain from every experience
	  • Go beyond your comfort zone

7. Demonstrate ethical and moral orientation.
  • Serve as a positive role model
  • Do not be judgmental
  • Foster personal development
	7. Demonstrate self-discipline in accepted responsibilities.

8. Bolster and affirm talents.	8. Hone time-management skills.
9. Advise the mentee about expectations and evaluation (i.e., research project-related, performance-related).	9. Demonstrate gratitude and respect.
10. Periodically re-evaluate the relationship.	10. Recognize that "the road to success is always under construction." The quest is never over.

Source: Nicholas G. Popovich, PhD, Associate Dean for Professional Development, University of Illinois at Chicago College of Pharmacy.

Research Proposal Guide

DEVELOPING A RESEARCH PROPOSAL

What are the components of a research proposal?

1. Title
2. Abstract
3. Introduction
4. Methods
5. Results (pending)
6. Conclusions (pending)
7. References

A well-planned and well-constructed research proposal will develop into your research manuscript.

Why is the TITLE important?

A properly constructed title will allow you to capture the reader's attention. It should be concise yet descriptive.

What is an ABSTRACT and what is its function?

- An abstract is a brief summary of the study described in the manuscript.
- It is usually limited to 200–300 words.
- An abstract introduces the reader to your paper; consider it the first impression, and make it a good one!

Questions to ask yourself when developing an ABSTRACT:

Are the objectives clearly stated?

Is the description of methods understandable?

Are the statistical tests used adequately described?

Are the results presented in sufficient detail to support the conclusions?

Are sound conclusions being made? Are they clearly presented?

Are there any practical implications of the information?

What does the INTRODUCTION include?

- Background, significance, and preliminary studies regarding your research topic
  - Includes an overview of the research literature on your topic
  - Describes the significance of your study
- The purpose of the study
  - What is the research question you are addressing? AND, why are you addressing it?
- Explains research question/research hypothesis
- Identifies the objectives of the study
  - Primary objectives
  - Secondary objectives

A well-executed manuscript leads to publications!

What does the METHODS section contain?

- Study design
  - What type of research are you conducting? Prospective? Retrospective? Survey-based?
  - What are the study sites? Is it single-center or multicenter?
- Study sample
  - What are your inclusion and exclusion criteria?
  - What is your procedure/protocol?
- Ethical considerations
  - How do you plan to maintain confidentiality?
  - How do you plan to manage your data?

- Statistical analysis
  - What are the statistical tests you will use to analyze your data?

What about the RESULTS and CONCLUSIONS?

- Results and conclusions should be marked as pending in a research proposal, as you will not have implemented your project.

What format do I use for REFERENCING?

- In general, use the AMA style of referencing. Ask your research mentor for more specifics.

Are there RESEARCH PROPOSAL format guidelines?

- No specific page length/font
  - Write as many pages as necessary for you to describe your project and the details on how you plan to implement it
- Writing should be formal

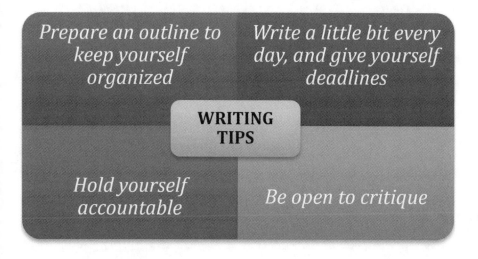

Prepare an outline to keep yourself organized

Write a little bit every day, and give yourself deadlines

WRITING TIPS

Hold yourself accountable

Be open to critique

APPENDIX E

Sample Research Proposal

To download Appendix E, please visit
http://media.pharmacist.com/AppendixE.docx

Perceptions of Fourth-Year Professional Students of a Capstone Research Project's Role in Pharmacy Job Attainment

Research students: Student or Resident Name, Credentials
Research mentor: Mentor Name, Credentials

RESEARCH PROPOSAL

INTRODUCTION

Background, Significance, and Preliminary Studies

Although most colleges of pharmacy in the United States require students to enroll in classes dedicated to biostatistics and research methods, it has been found that only approximately one-quarter of these schools require a research component in their curriculum.[1] According to guideline 23.4, the Accreditation Council for Pharmacy Education strongly encourages that research be incorporated into pharmacy education.[2] Capstone projects are research-based projects performed in the final year of the doctor of pharmacy curriculum to fulfill this guideline. A capstone research project is a fourth-year professional pharmacy student's endeavor to use all previous pharmaceutical and scientific knowledge learned didactically and through prior experiences.[3] Major components of capstone research projects may vary; some components that have been cited in the literature include project proposal or selection of a specific objective to be explored, institutional review board submission, analysis of collected data, and presentation of results in the form of a manuscript, poster, or both.[3–5] Pharmacy programs may also have varying components and time frames for completion of capstone research projects; however, in general the project is completed during the fourth professional year. Additionally, not all programs have a dedicated advanced practice experience (APPE) rotation allocated for students' work on the capstone research project.[4,5]

A required capstone research project not only provides fourth-year pharmacy students an opportunity to use critical thinking skills but also allows them to design and implement a research project from beginning to end. Students are required to work semi-independently with a faculty member or preceptor who serves as a research mentor to develop skills associated with research. These include performing a literature search, formulating a research question, and analyzing data for possible conclusions. In previous investigations of research mentors' perceptions of senior research projects, most preceptors have agreed that a senior research project is extremely beneficial and advantageous to pharmacy students.[4,5]

Similarly, pharmacy students have positive attitudes toward a required research project and believe that conducting a capstone research project is a fulfilling and valuable learning experience.[6] To date, no studies have investigated the types of skills students perceive they have obtained upon completing a capstone research project.

Performing research in the final year of a pharmacy program showcases the student's ability to use critical thinking skills, decipher medical literature, and apply findings of the research literature to enhance or develop evidence-based medicine practices.[6] This experience can prepare students for a fellowship or residency, in which research is a vital part of the students' postgraduate training. Kim and colleagues showed that 86.1% of students planning to undertake a fellowship or residency believe a capstone research experience makes them a more suitable candidate.[6] According to the American College of Clinical Pharmacy, required research is believed to "motivate students to pursue education and training beyond the PharmD degree."[6]

Currently, there are six colleges of pharmacy in Illinois, an increase from two in 2005. Two of the six programs have incorporated a required capstone research project into their curricula. With the increasing number of doctor of pharmacy graduates in the state, having research experience may enhance a student's resume in the eyes of potential employers or residency program directors and may increase the student's chances of being selected for interviews or employment.

With the saturation of the pharmacy job market in the Chicago area, attaining a position after graduation can be a challenge. The Aggregate Demand Index is a market analysis carried out monthly that determines the demand for pharmacists in various states and regions. It uses a numerical scale where 5 = high demand, difficult to fill open positions; 4 = moderate demand, some difficulty filling open positions; 3 = demand in balance with supply; 2 = demand is less than the pharmacist supply available; and 1 = demand is much less than the pharmacist supply available. Over the past five years, there has been a considerable decline in the demand for pharmacists in Illinois. In March 2008, the demand index was 4.13, followed by 3.5 in 2009, 3.22 in 2010, 3.11 in 2011, and finally 3.13 in 2012. As of March 2012, Illinois is classified as having a balanced supply and demand of pharmacists, in contrast to March 2008 when there was a moderate demand and some difficulty filling open positions.[7] With the additional doctor of pharmacy programs in the Chicago area, this index may not be applicable to the region, which could potentially have an oversupply of pharmacists in the near future, if it does not already. Therefore, it is essential that students' perceptions of a capstone research project increasing their marketability for attaining a job upon graduation be investigated.

OBJECTIVES

As doctor of pharmacy graduates continue to enter the workforce in Illinois, they must differentiate themselves from other applicants, and conducting a required research project in their final professional year may provide an opportunity to do this. The primary objective of this study is to investigate whether conducting a capstone research project makes fourth-year doctor of pharmacy candidates more confident in attaining a job position upon graduation. Secondary objectives are to determine the types of skills pharmacy students perceive they obtain from performing a capstone project, to determine their level of comfort with their perceived skills, and to ascertain whether pharmacy students feel they can use their perceived skills to enhance their future practice as pharmacists.

METHODS

Research Methods and Design

This study will be conducted at three colleges of pharmacy in Illinois, one each in an urban, suburban, and rural setting. All three colleges have fourth-year pharmacy students enrolled in APPE rotations. Two of the colleges require a capstone research project as part of their pharmacy curriculum while one college does not. Thus, differences in student perceptions in the programs that require a capstone research project and the program that does not will be analyzed via two different questionnaires.

Two student pharmacists will coordinate with staff at all three colleges to administer the surveys. Only those students who are in their fourth year of pharmacy school with anticipated graduation occurring in spring 2013 will be included. The survey will take approximately 10 minutes to complete. It consists of five sections, including demographics, general capstone research project questions, perceptions of a capstone research project, perceptions of skills gained by performing a capstone research project, and job attainment as it relates to capstone projects. Most questions use a 4-point Likert scale (A = strongly agree, B = agree, C = disagree, D = strongly disagree).

Data will be collected and analyzed with SPSS Version 18 using chi-square analysis and descriptive statistics. All data will be anonymous and maintained confidentially.

TIMELINE

12 MONTHS

Activity	Month
IRB approval	June–July 2014
Administration of survey	August–September 2014
Formulation of results and statistical analysis	October–December 2014
Finalization of results	February 2015
Abstract submission for poster presentation	March 2015
Poster presentation	May 2015
Write manuscript for publication	June 2016

REFERENCES

1. Murphy J, Slack M, Buesen K, et al. Research-related coursework and research experiences in doctor of pharmacy programs. *Am J Pharm Educ.* 2007;71(6):1–7.
2. Accreditation standards and guidelines for the professional program in pharmacy leading to the doctor of pharmacy degree. *ACPE.* 2011;40.
3. Wuller CA. A capstone advanced pharmacy practice experience in research. *Am J Pharm Educ.* 2010;74(10):1–7.
4. Kao D, Suchanek Hudmon K, Corelli R. Evaluation of a required senior research project in a doctor of pharmacy curriculum. *Am J Pharm Educ.* 2011;75(1):1–7.
5. Murphy J. Faculty attitudes toward required evaluative projects for doctor of pharmacy candidates. *Am J Pharm Educ.* 1997;61:73-78.
6. Kim S, Whittington J, Nguyen L, et al. Pharmacy students' perceptions of a required senior research project. *Am J Pharm Educ.* 2010;74(10):1–7.
7. Aggregate Demand Index. Pharmacy Manpower Project Inc. www.pharmacymanpower.com/index.jsp. Accessed June 7, 2014.

Steps in the Research Process

Step	Research Process
1.	Identify the study question. • Develop a research proposal
2.	Determine the study approach/study design. • Submit an application to the IRB
3.	Collect data.
4.	Analyze data.
5.	Report findings. • Poster/platform presentation • Manuscript submission

Sample Survey with Codebook and Database

Survey

1. What is your age? _____ years old

2. What is your gender?
   a. Male = 1
   b. Female = 2

3. What is your race/ethnicity?
   a. African-American/Black = 1
   b. American Indian/Alaskan Native = 2
   c. Asian American = 3
   d. Latino/Hispanic = 4
   e. Native Hawaiian/Pacific Islander = 5
   f. Caucasian = 6
   g. Other (specify) = 7

4. Which of the following health conditions do you have? (Circle all that apply):
   a. Diabetes (Yes = 1, No = 2)
   b. High blood pressure (Yes = 1, No = 2)
   c. High cholesterol (Yes = 1, No = 2)
   d. Depression (Yes = 1, No = 2)
   e. Menopause (Yes = 1, No = 2)
   f. Osteoporosis (Yes = 1, No = 2)
   g. Migraine headache (Yes = 1, No = 2)
   h. Anxiety (Yes = 1, No = 2)
   i. Insomnia (Yes = 1, No = 2)

5. Have you ever owned a fish tank or an indoor aquarium?
   a. Yes = 1 (If Yes, skip to # 7)
   b. No = 2

6. If "No" (in question # 5), are you interested in having a fish tank or an indoor aquarium?
   a. Yes = 1
   b. No = 2

7. Do you enjoy gardening?
   a. Yes = 1
   b. No = 2

8. Do you prepare your own beverages or meals (for example, tea) at this facility?
   a. Yes = 1
   b. No = 2

9. Do you sometimes eat healthy, fresh produce or herbs brought in from outside the facility (if you reside here)?
   a. Yes = 1
   b. No = 2
   c. Not applicable = 3

10. How many times a day on average do you eat fresh, healthful produce or herbs?
    a. 0 times = 0
    b. 1 time = 1
    c. 2 times = 2
    d. 3 times = 3
    e. More than 3 times = 4

Codebook

Question	Code
1. What is your age? _____ years old	age
2. What is your gender? a. Male = 1 b. Female = 2	gen

Question	Code
3. What is your race/ethnicity? 　a. African-American/Black = 1 　b. American Indian/Alaskan Native = 2 　c. Asian American = 3 　d. Latino/Hispanic = 4 　e. Native Hawaiian/Pacific Islander = 5 　f. Caucasian = 6 　g. Other (specify) = 7	race g. racespec
4. Which of the following health conditions do you have? (Circle all that apply): 　a. Diabetes (Yes = 1, No = 2) 　b. High blood pressure (Yes = 1, No = 2) 　c. High cholesterol (Yes = 1, No = 2) 　d. Depression (Yes = 1, No = 2) 　e. Menopause (Yes = 1, No = 2) 　f. Osteoporosis (Yes = 1, No = 2) 　g. Migraine headache (Yes = 1, No = 2) 　h. Anxiety (Yes = 1, No = 2) 　i. Insomnia (Yes = 1, No = 2)	Health cond
5. Have you ever owned a fish tank or an indoor aquarium? 　a. Yes = 1 (If Yes, skip to # 7) 　b. No = 2	tank
6. If "No" (in question # 5), are you interested in having a fish tank or an indoor aquarium? 　a. Yes = 1 　b. No = 2	tankno
7. Do you enjoy gardening? 　a. Yes = 1 　b. No = 2	gard
8. Do you prepare your own beverages or meals (for example, tea) at this facility? 　a. Yes = 1 　b. No = 2	bevmea

Question	Code
9. Do you sometimes eat healthy, fresh produce or herbs brought in from outside the facility (if you reside here)? a. Yes = 1 b. No = 2 c. Not applicable = 3	fresh
10. How many times a day on average do you eat fresh, healthful produce or herbs? a. 0 times = 0 b. 1 time = 1 c. 2 times = 2 d. 3 times = 3 e. More than 3 times = 4	freshavg

Database

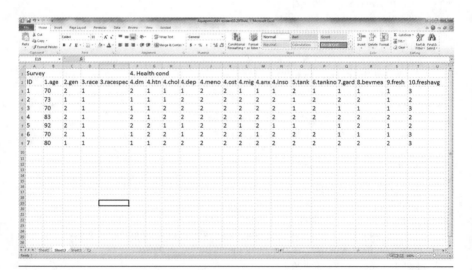

Sample Abstract

Perceptions of Fourth-Year Professional Students of a Capstone Research Project's Role in Pharmacy Job Attainment

Objective: To investigate students' perceptions of a capstone research requirement, their perceived comfort levels with research skills, and their confidence in future job attainment.

Methods: Fourth professional year pharmacy students at three colleges of pharmacy completed a questionnaire. Data were analyzed using chi-square analysis and descriptive statistics.

Results: A total of 219 surveys were received, yielding a 70% response rate. Approximately 40% of students were required to complete a research project (capstone); 60% did not (non-capstone). Capstone students reported improved comfort with all perceived research skills; 9 out of 10 skills showed a significant increase in comfort ($P < 0.001$). Approximately 72% in the capstone group and 58% in the non-capstone group believed skills learned in research would enhance future practice ($P < 0.01$). Fifty-one percent of capstone students felt more confident in job attainment after graduation ($P = 0.19$).

Conclusion: Students perceive a capstone research project to be beneficial with regard to skills, marketability, and enhancing future practice.

APPENDIX I

Sample Posters

To download the three sample posters in Appendix I, please visit
http://media.pharmacist.com/SamplePoster1.pptx
http://media.pharmacist.com/SamplePoster2.ppt
http://media.pharmacist.com/SamplePoster3.ppt

Perceptions of Fourth-Year Professional Students of a Capstone Research Project's Role in Pharmacy Job Attainment

Author Names

Name of College of Pharmacy

Background and Introduction

- One quarter of all colleges of pharmacy in the United States require a research component in their curriculum.[1]
- According to Accreditation Standards Guideline 23.4, the Accreditation Council for Pharmacy Education strongly encourages that research be incorporated into pharmacy education.[2]
- A capstone research project is a fourth-year pharmacy student's endeavor in research intended to use all previous pharmaceutical and scientific knowledge gained in the classroom and through prior experiences.[3]
- **Components of a capstone research project:**
  - Working with a research mentor   • Carrying out the project from start to finish
  - Selecting a specific objective   • Formulating a manuscript
  - Performing a literature search   • Creating a poster
- Previous investigations regarding perceptions of senior research projects show:
  - **Mentors:** Agree that a senior research project is extremely beneficial and advantageous to pharmacy students.[4,5]
  - **Pharmacy students:** Have positive attitudes toward a required research project and believe doing a capstone project is a fulfilling/valuable learning experience.[6]
- There are six colleges of pharmacy in Illinois, an increase from two in 2005.
- The Aggregate Demand Index is a monthly market analysis that determines the demand for pharmacists in various states and regions.[7]
  - 5= high demand
  - 4= moderate demand
  - 3= demand = supply
  - 2= demand < supply
  - 1= demand << supply

Year	Aggregate Demand Index
2008	4.13
2009	3.5
2010	3.22
2011	3.11
2012	3.13

- As doctor of pharmacy graduates continue to enter the workforce in Illinois, they must differentiate themselves from other applicants.
- Conducting a required research project in their final professional year may provide an opportunity for this to occur.[7]

Objectives

Primary Objective:
- To determine if conducting a fourth-professional-year research project (capstone) makes pharmacy students more confident in attaining a job position upon graduation.

Secondary Objectives:
- To determine the types of skills pharmacy students perceive they obtained from performing a capstone project.
- To determine the pharmacy students' level of comfort with their perceived research skills.
- To determine if pharmacy students feel they can use their perceived skills to enhance their future practice.

Methods

- A paper questionnaire was administered at CSU-COP & MWU-CCP; an electronic survey was administered at SIUE-COP.
- Two of the colleges required a capstone project, and one college did not.
- Only students in their fourth year of pharmacy school with anticipated graduation occurring on spring 2013 were included.
- The survey consisted of five sections:
  - Demographics, General capstone research project questions, Perceptions of a capstone research project, Perceptions of skills gained by performing a capstone research project, and Job attainment
- Most questions used a 4-point Likert scale.
- Data were collected and analyzed with SPSS software, using chi-square analysis and descriptive statistics.

Results

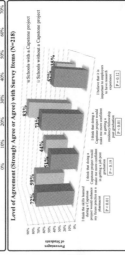

Student Demographics (N=219)

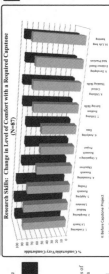

Level of Agreement (Strongly Agree or Agree) with Survey Items (N=218)

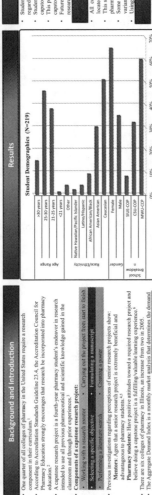

Research Skills: Change in Level of Comfort with a Required Capstone (N=87)

Implications

- Students reported an increase in comfort level when performing a capstone project in regard to skills they perceived they had obtained.
- Students who elect to apply for postgraduate training may consider conducting a capstone research project to improve their confidence in obtaining a position.
- This provides increased support for colleges of pharmacy considering incorporating a capstone research project into their curriculum.
- Future studies may determine whether employers or residency program directors rank research experience as a priority when selecting candidates for interview.

Limitations

- All colleges of pharmacy in Illinois were not assessed; those that participated were located in three different geographic regions – suburban, urban, and rural.
- This study may not be as applicable to areas where there is still a demand for pharmacists.
- Some students were at different points in their capstone research project, which led to a variance in perceptions.
- Using an electronic survey at SIUE-COP resulted in a decreased response rate.

Conclusions

- Fourth-professional-year students at universities with a required research component became more comfortable with all of the capstone research-associated skills upon completing or during work on a required capstone research project.
- Approximately 51% of students with a required capstone research project and 44% of those without a required capstone research project believed the skills learned from a capstone research project would help them better attain jobs as pharmacists.
- About 72% of students who completed a required capstone research project and 59% who did not believed that the skills learned during a capstone research project would enhance their future practice as pharmacists.
- Thus, students perceive a capstone research project to be beneficial in terms of skills, marketability, and enhancing their future practice.

Acknowledgments

The authors would like to acknowledge Drs. Doe and Smith for their contributions with statistical analysis in this study.

Disclosures

- The authors have no potential conflicts of interest to disclose.

References

1. Murphy J, Slack M, Boesen K, et al. Research related coursework and research experiences in doctor of pharmacy programs. *Am J Pharm Educ.* 2007;71(6):1-7.
2. Accreditation standards and guidelines for the professional program in pharmacy leading to the doctor of pharmacy degree. *ACPE.* 2011:1-99.
3. Waller CA. A capstone advanced pharmacy practice experience in research. *Am J Pharm Educ.* 2010;74(10):1-7.
4. Kao D, Suchanek Hudmon K, Corelli R. Evaluation of a required senior research project in a doctor of pharmacy curriculum. *Am J Pharm Educ.* 2011;75(1):1-7.
5. Murphy J. Faculty and student attitudes toward required evaluative projects for doctor of pharmacy candidates. *Am J Pharm Educ.* 1997;61:73-78.
6. Kim S, Willett R, Noguera J, Nguyen L, et al. Pharmacy students' perceptions of a required senior research project. *Am J Pharm Educ.* 2010;74(10):1-7.
7. Aggregate Demand Index. Pharmacy Manpower Project Inc. www.pharmacymanpower.com/index.jsp. Accessed June 7, 2012.

For more information contact:
Name 1, PharmD Candidate   Name 2, PharmD Candidate
email address   email address
                          Mentor Name, PharmD
                          email address

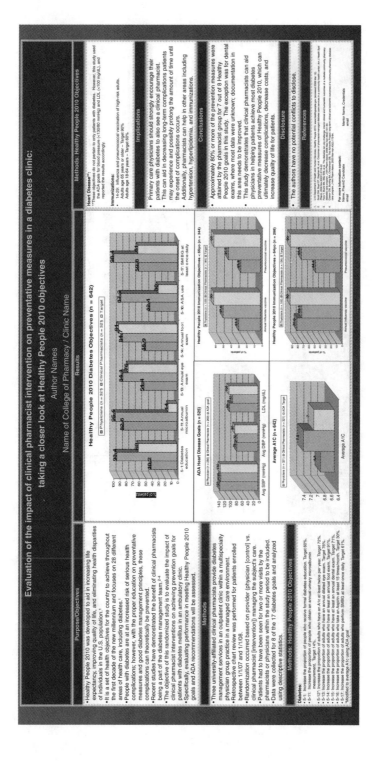

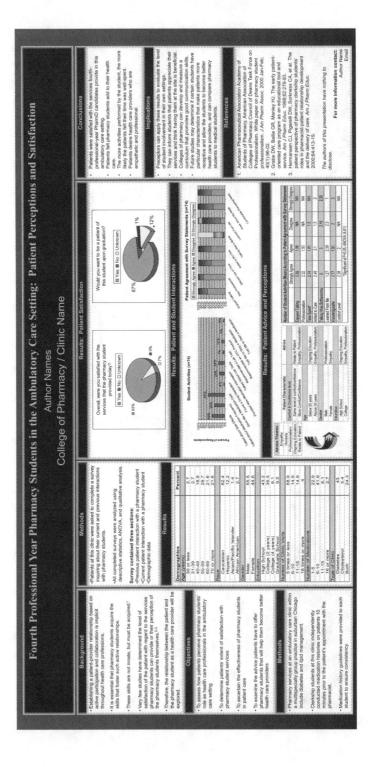

APPENDIX J

Sample Poster Template

To download the poster template, please visit
http://media.pharmacist.com/PosterTemplate.pptx

Insert
Logo
Here

Insert
Logo
Here

Title

Authors

Name of College of Pharmacy or Practice Site

Introduction

• This section is for the introduction of your study. It includes background studies and the purpose and significance of your study. (Choose font size no less than 24). Include objectives toward the end of this section.

• *NOTE: The size of all of the text boxes and the appearance of the sections can be adjusted and modified to fit your poster's needs. You are not restricted to this exact layout. The colors of the poster, however, must remain the same.*

Methods

• Write your methods here. Include comments on the study design, procedure/protocols, institutional approval, and statistical methods used.

Results

• Results/data should be depicted visually using graphs, charts, tables, diagrams, etc. Attempt to strike a good balance between the layout of tables/figures/charts and the text of this poster. All posters must have visual appeal and must include visual formats other than plain text. Be creative!

Discussion

• Discuss your overall impressions of the study here. Based on your data, what are the strengths, future implications, and limitations of the study?

Conclusions

• Write a summary of your overall conclusions of the study here.
• *NOTE: All boxes should line up evenly and align properly once you are finished with the content of your poster. Complete this task last.*

References

• References can appear in a smaller font size than the rest of the poster (no less than size 18). Be sure to cite your references within the introduction.

APPENDIX K

Sample Manuscript Template

To download the manuscript template, please visit
http://media.pharmacist.com/ManuscriptTemplate.docx

The title should accurately, clearly, and concisely reflect the emphasis and content of the paper. The title must be brief and grammatically correct. (Delete this italicized section when done.)

THE TITLE OF YOUR MANUSCRIPT GOES HERE

Student Name 1, PharmD Candidate[1]; Resident Name 2, PharmD[1]
Mentor Name 1, Credentials[1,2]; Mentor Name 2, Credentials[1,2]

[1] Name of College of Pharmacy, City; [2]Mentor Affiliation, City

> Insert College or
> Clinic Logo
> Here

All manuscripts must be accompanied by an abstract. The abstract should briefly state the problem or purpose of the research, indicate the theoretical or experimental plan used, summarize the principal findings, and point out the major conclusions. Limit the abstract to 300 words, and use a font size of 9. (Delete this italicized section when done.)
Background:
Methods:
Results:
Conclusions:

This section here will begin your introduction. Discuss background literature evidence and the rationale for and significance of conducting your study. Font should be size 10.

(FYI: Always leave a space between section titles. Titles should be capitalized and font size 11. Writing and subtitles should be font size 10). (Delete this section when done.)

OBJECTIVES

Describe the objectives of the study in this section.

METHODS

Study Design and Procedures
Describe the study design and associated procedures in this section.

Endpoints
Describe endpoints if applicable.

Statistical Analysis
Describe statistical methods used in the study.

RESULTS

Describe the results of the study in this section. Tables and figures should be placed ideally near where you are describing that particular section in the text. Try to find a good balance between the layout of tables/figures and text throughout the manuscript. Note: It is always a good idea to develop your results tables first, and then work on describing them in the text.

Note: All tables/figures should be numbered sequentially. Abbreviations needing further explanation should be placed as a footnote underneath the table or figure. Examples are provided below. (Delete this italicized section when done.)

TABLE 1: Baseline Characteristics (N=53)

Age (years)	
Mean±SD (Range)	75.23±2.321 (63–85)
Gender [N(%)]*	
Males	41 (77.4)
Females	12 (22.6)

*If you needed to explain something further regarding gender, place additional info here.

FIGURE 1: Age Groups with Hypertension (N=73)

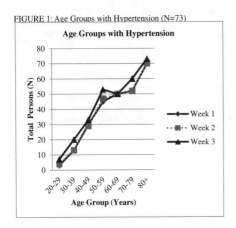

DISCUSSION

Consider this section the "author's voice." As the author, you should speak of your overall impressions of the study, discussing key findings, limitations, and future implications. Start with the key findings of the study. This is also a good opportunity to link similarities or differences in the results you obtained back to the background literature. Then, discuss your thoughts on limitations of the study. Finally, include a section on future implications. This involves describing your thoughts on studies that can be conducted in the future that may complement or enhance the work you have completed thus far.

CONCLUSIONS

Your overall summary of the conclusions or major findings of your study (based on the data) should be written here.

ACKNOWLEDGMENTS

Here, you acknowledge people for their contributions to your research project. Note: Co-authors are not acknowledged.

REFERENCES

Should be very small font size 8. (Delete this italicized section when done.)

1. Reference 1
2. Reference 2

Index